Interventional Head and Neck Imaging

Guest Editor

DHEERAJ GANDHI, MD

NEUROIMAGING CLINICS OF NORTH AMERICA

www.neuroimaging.theclinics.com

Consulting Editor
SURESH K. MUKHERJI, MD

May 2009 • Volume 19 • Number 2

SAUNDERS an imprint of ELSEVIER, Inc.

W.B. SAUNDERS COMPANY
A Division of Elsevier Inc.

1600 John F. Kennedy Boulevard • Suite 1800 • Philadelphia, Pennsylvania 19103-2899

http://www.theclinics.com

NEUROIMAGING CLINICS OF NORTH AMERICA Volume 19, Number 2
May 2009 ISSN 1052-5149, ISBN 13: 978-1-4377-0503-4, ISBN 10: 1-4377-0503-0

Editor: Donald Mumford

Photocopying
Single photocopies of single articles may be made for personal use as allowed by national copyright laws. Permission of the Publisher and payment of a fee is required for all other photocopying, including multiple or systematic copying, copying for advertising or promotional purposes, resale, and all forms of document delivery. Special rates are available for educational institutions that wish to make photocopies for non-profit educational classroom use. For information on how to seek permission visit www.elsevier.com/permissions or call: (+44) 1865 843830 (UK)/(+1) 215 239 3804 (USA).

Derivative Works
Subscribers may reproduce tables of contents or prepare lists of articles including abstracts for internal circulation within their institutions. Permission of the Publisher is required for resale or distribution outside the institution. Permission of the Publisher is required for all other derivative works, including compilations and translations (please consult www.elsevier.com/permissions).

Electronic Storage or Usage
Permission of the Publisher is required to store or use electronically any material contained in this journal, including any article or part of an article (please consult www.elsevier.com/permissions). Except as outlined above, no part of this publication may be reproduced, stored in a retrieval system or transmitted in any form or by any means, electronic, mechanical, photocopying, recording or otherwise, without prior written permission of the Publisher.

Notice
No responsibility is assumed by the Publisher for any injury and/or damage to persons or property as a matter of products liability, negligence or otherwise, or from any use or operation of any methods, products, instructions or ideas contained in the material herein. Because of rapid advances in the medical sciences, in particular, independent verification of diagnoses and drug dosages should be made.

Although all advertising material is expected to conform to ethical (medical) standards, inclusion in this publication does not constitute a guarantee or endorsement of the quality or value of such product or of the claims made of it by its manufacturer.

Neuroimaging Clinics of North America (ISSN 1052-5149) is published quarterly by Elsevier Inc., 360 Park Avenue South, New York, NY 10010-1710. Months of issue are February, May, August, and November. Business and editorial offices: 1600 John F. Kennedy Blvd., Suite 1800, Philadelphia, PA 19103-2899. Business and editorial offices: 6277 Sea Harbor Drive, Orlando, FL 32887-4800. Periodicals postage paid at New York, NY, and additional mailing offices. Subscription prices are USD 264 per year for US individuals, USD 407 per year for US institutions, USD 135 per year for US students and residents, USD 305 per year for Canadian individuals, USD 510 per year for Canadian institutions, USD 388 per year for international individuals, USD 510 per year for international institutions and USD 194 per year for Canadian and foreign students and residents. To receive student/resident rate, orders must be accompanied by name of affiliated institution, date of term, and the *signature* of program/residency coordinator on institution letterhead. Orders will be billed at individual rate until proof of status is received. Foreign air speed delivery is included in all *Clinics* subscription prices. All prices are subject to change without notice. POSTMASTER: Send address changes to *Neuroimaging Clinics of North America*, Elsevier Periodicals Customer Service, 11830 Westline Industrial Drive, St. Louis, MO 63146. Customer Service (orders, claims, online, change of address): Elsevier Periodicals Customer Service, 11830 Westline Industrial Drive, St. Louis, MO 63146. Tel: 1-800-654-2452 (U.S. and Canada); 314-453-7041 (outside U.S. and Canada). Fax: 314-453-5170. E-mail: journalscustomerservice-usa@elsevier.com (for print support); journalsonlinesupport-usa@elsevier.com (for online support).

Reprints. For copies of 100 or more of articles in this publication, please contact the Commercial Reprints Department, Elsevier Inc., 360 Park Avenue South, New York, NY 10010-1710. Tel.: 212-633-3812; Fax: 212-462-1935; E-mail: reprints@elsevier.com.

Neuroimaging Clinics of North America is covered by *Excerpta Medical/EMBASE,* the RSNA Index of Imaging Literature, *MEDLINE/PubMed (Index Medicus),* MEDLINE/MEDLARS, SciSearch, Research Alert, and Neuroscience Citation Index.

Cover image © Lydia Gregg 2009.

Printed and bound by CPI Group (UK) Ltd, Croydon, CR0 4YY

Transferred to Digital Print 2011

GOAL STATEMENT

The goal of *Neuroimaging Clinics of North America* is to keep practicing radiologists and radiology residents up to date with current clinical practice in radiology by providing timely articles reviewing the state of the art in patient care.

ACCREDITATION

The *Neuroimaging Clinics of North America* is planned and implemented in accordance with the Essential Areas and Policies of the Accreditation Council for Continuing Medical Education (ACCME) through the joint sponsorship of the University of Virginia School of Medicine and Elsevier. The University of Virginia School of Medicine is accredited by the ACCME to provide continuing medical education for physicians.

The University of Virginia School of Medicine designates this educational activity for a maximum of 15 *AMA PRA Category 1 Credits*™ for each issue, 60 credits per year. Physicians should only claim credit commensurate with the extent of their participation in the activity.

The American Medical Association has determined that physicians not licensed in the US who participate in this CME activity are eligible for a maximum of 15 *AMA PRA Category 1 Credits*™ for each issue, 60 credits per year.

Credit can be earned by reading the text material, taking the CME examination online at http://www.theclinics.com/home/cme, and completing the evaluation. After taking the test, you will be required to review any and all incorrect answers. Following completion of the test and evaluation, your credit will be awarded and you may print your certificate.

FACULTY DISCLOSURE/CONFLICT OF INTEREST

The University of Virginia School of Medicine, as an ACCME accredited provider, endorses and strives to comply with the Accreditation Council for Continuing Medical Education (ACCME) Standards of Commercial Support, Commonwealth of Virginia statutes, University of Virginia policies and procedures, and associated federal and private regulations and guidelines on the need for disclosure and monitoring of proprietary and financial interests that may affect the scientific integrity and balance of content delivered in continuing medical education activities under our auspices.

The University of Virginia School of Medicine requires that all CME activities accredited through this institution be developed independently and be scientifically rigorous, balanced and objective in the presentation/discussion of its content, theories and practices.

All authors/editors participating in an accredited CME activity are expected to disclose to the readers relevant financial relationships with commercial entities occurring within the past 12 months (such as grants or research support, employee, consultant, stock holder, member of speakers bureau, etc.). The University of Virginia School of Medicine will employ appropriate mechanisms to resolve potential conflicts of interest to maintain the standards of fair and balanced education to the reader. Questions about specific strategies can be directed to the Office of Continuing Medical Education, University of Virginia School of Medicine, Charlottesville, Virginia.

The faculty and staff of the University of Virginia Office of Continuing Medical Education have no financial affiliations to disclose.

The authors/editors listed below have identified no professional/financial affiliations for themselves or their spouse/partner:
Ahmad I Alomari, MD; Sameer A. Ansari, MD, PhD; Gulraiz Chaudry, MD; David J. Choi, MD, PhD; DeWitte T. Cross, III, MD; Dheeraj Gandhi, MD (Guest Editor); Lydia Gregg, MA; Sanjay Gupta, MD; William Holloway, MD; Mohannad Ibrahim, MD; Sudhir Kathuria, MD; Avi Mazumdar, MD; Jonathan B. McHugh, MD; Donald Mumford (Acquiring Editor); Kieran Murphy, MB, BCh; Darren B. Orbach, MD, PhD; Diego San Millán Ruiz, MD; Gaurang Shah, MD; Isaac C. Wu, MD; and Gerald Wyse, MB, BCh.

The authors listed below have identified the following professional/financial affiliations for themselves or their spouse/partner:
Colin P. Derdeyn, MD serves on the Advisory Committee for W.L. Gore and Associates and owns stock in nFocus, Inc.
Phillipe Gailloud, MD is a consultant for Cordis Neurovascular and owns stock in ArtVentive.
Joseph J. Gemmete, MD is a consultant for and owns stock in CORDIS.
H. Hong, MD serves on the Speakers Bureau for Boston Scientific and Covidien
Christopher J. Moran, MD is an industry funded research/investigator, consultant, and serves on the Speakers Bureau for Boston Scientific/Target and is a consultant and serves on the Speakers Bureau for eU3.
Suresh K. Mukherji, MD (Consulting Editor) is a consultant for Philips Medical Systems and GE.
Hermant Parmar, MD is an industry funded research/investigator for Bayer Healthcare.

Disclosure of Discussion of Non-FDA Approved Uses for Pharmaceutical Products and/or Medical Devices.
The University of Virginia School of Medicine, as an ACCME provider, requires that all faculty presenters identify and disclose any off-label uses for pharmaceutical and medical device products. The University of Virginia School of Medicine recommends that each physician fully review all the available data on new products or procedures prior to clinical use.

TO ENROLL

To enroll in the Neuroimaging Clinics of North America Continuing Medical Education program, call customer service at 1-800-654-2452 or sign up online at *http://www.theclinics.com/home/cme*. The CME program is available to subscribers for an additional annual fee of USD 175.

Neuroimaging Clinics of North America

THE CLINICS ARE NOW AVAILABLE ONLINE!

Access your subscription at:
www.theclinics.com

Contributors

CONSULTING EDITOR

SURESH K. MUKHERJI, MD
Professor and Chief of Neuroradiology and
Head and Neck Radiology; Professor of
Radiology, Otolaryngology Head Neck Surgery
and Radiation Oncology, University of
Michigan Health System, Ann Arbor, Michigan

GUEST EDITOR

DHEERAJ GANDHI, MD
Assistant Professor of Radiology, Neurology,
and Neurosurgery, Johns Hopkins University
and Hospitals, Division of Interventional
Neuroradiology, Baltimore, Maryland

AUTHORS

AHMAD I. ALOMARI, MD
Assistant Professor of Radiology, Division of
Interventional Radiology, Children's Hospital
Boston, Harvard Medical School, Boston,
Massachusetts

SAMEER A. ANSARI, MD, PhD
Assistant Professor; Director,
Neurointerventional Service, Diagnostic
and Interventional Neuroradiology,
Departments of Radiology, Neurology, and
Surgery, University of Chicago Medical Center,
Chicago, Illinois

GULRAIZ CHAUDRY, MD
Instructor in Radiology, Division of
Interventional Radiology, Children's Hospital
Boston, Harvard Medical School, Boston,
Massachusetts

DAVID J. CHOI, MD, PhD
Division of Neuroradiology, Brigham and
Women's Hospital, Harvard Medical School,
Boston, Massachusetts

DeWITTE T. CROSS, III, MD
Mallinckrodt Institute of Radiology,
Washington University School of Medicine;
Department of Neurological Surgery,
Washington University School of Medicine,
St. Louis, Missouri

COLIN P. DERDEYN, MD
Mallinckrodt Institute of Radiology,
Washington University School of Medicine;
Department of Neurology, Washington
University School of Medicine; Department of
Neurological Surgery, Washington University
School of Medicine, St. Louis, Missouri

PHILIPPE GAILLOUD, MD
Division of Interventional Neuroradiology, The
Johns Hopkins Hospital, Baltimore, Maryland

DHEERAJ GANDHI, MD
Assistant Professor of Radiology, Neurology,
and Neurosurgery, Johns Hopkins University
and Hospitals, Division of Interventional
Neuroradiology, Baltimore, Maryland

JOSEPH J. GEMMETE, MD
Assistant Professor, Division of Interventional
Neuroradiology, Department of Radiology,
University of Michigan Health System,
Ann Arbor, Michigan

LYDIA GREGG, MA
Division of Interventional Neuroradiology,
The Johns Hopkins Hospital, Baltimore,
Maryland

SANJAY GUPTA, MD
Associate Professor, Department
of Diagnostic Radiology, The University of
Texas M.D. Anderson Cancer Center,
Houston, Texas

WILLIAM HOLLOWAY, MD
Mallinckrodt Institute of Radiology,
Washington University School of Medicine,
St. Louis, Missouri

H. HONG, MD
Assistant Professor, Division of Interventional
Radiology, Department of Radiology, Johns
Hopkins Medical Institutions, Baltimore,
Maryland

MOHANNAD IBRAHIM, MD
Department of Radiology, University of
Michigan Health System, Ann Arbor, Michigan

SUDHIR KATHURIA, MD
Division of Interventional Neuroradiology,
Department of Radiology, Johns
Hopkins University and Hospitals, Baltimore,
Maryland

AVI MAZUMDAR, MD
Mallinckrodt Institute of Radiology,
Washington University School of Medicine;
Department of Neurology, Washington
University School of Medicine, St. Louis,
Missouri; Department of Interventional
Neuroradiology, Central DuPage Hospital,
Winfield, Illinois

JONATHAN McHUGH, MD
Assistant Professor, Department of Pathology,
University of Michigan Health System,
Ann Arbor, Michigan

CHRISTOPHER J. MORAN, MD
Mallinckrodt Institute of Radiology,
Washington University School of Medicine;
Department of Neurological Surgery,
Washington University School of Medicine,
St. Louis, Missouri

KIERAN MURPHY, MB, BCh
Professor and Vice Chair; Director of Research,
University of Toronto Medical Imaging,
Toronto, Ontario, Canada; Deputy Chief,
Medical Imaging, University Health Network,
MSH and Woman's Hospital

DARREN B. ORBACH, MD, PhD
Assistant Professor of Radiology, Division of
Neurointerventional Radiology, Children's
Hospital Boston, Brigham and Women's
Hospital, Harvard Medical School, Boston,
Massachusetts

HEMANT PARMAR, MD
Department of Radiology, University of
Michigan Health System, Ann Arbor, Michigan

DIEGO SAN MILLÁN RUIZ, MD
Division of Interventional Neuroradiology, The
Johns Hopkins Hospital, Baltimore, Maryland

GAURANG SHAH, MD
Department of Radiology, University of
Michigan Health System, Ann Arbor, Michigan

ISAAC C. WU, MD
Neuroradiology Division, Brigham and
Women's Hospital, Harvard Medical School,
Boston, Massachusetts

GERALD WYSE, MB, BCh
Instructor, Division of Interventional
Neuroradiology, Department of Radiology,
Johns Hopkins University, Baltimore, Maryland

Contents

Dheeraj Gandhi, Sudhir Kathuria, Sameer A. Ansari, Gaurang Shah, and Joseph J. Gemmete

Recent technologic advances including multidetector CT, dynamic CT angiography, high-field MR imaging, four-dimensional MR angiography, and physiologic studies, such as perfusion imaging, have revolutionized the imaging work-up of head, neck, and skull base lesions. These techniques not only provide accurate diagnostic information, but also help plan endovascular therapy. The future holds great promise for interventional neuroradiologists because excellent imaging tools are becoming available that are capable of providing morphologic, hemodynamic, and physiologic information. Furthermore, availability of faster, real-time guidance systems and hybrid systems improves the ability to perform procedures not only in a rapid and safe manner but also with great precision.

Sanjay Gupta

Use of image-guidance allows safe and precise percutaneous placement of needles for various diagnostic and therapeutic procedures in the head and neck region. This review describes the anatomy relevant to safe-access route planning and the techniques, advantages, and limitations associated with various approaches used for percutaneous needle placement in different head and neck regions. Subzygomatic, retromandibular, paramaxillary, submastoid, transoral, and posterior approaches can be used for percutaneous access in the suprahyoid head and neck region, including skull base and upper cervical vertebrae. In the infrahyoid portion of the neck and for lower cervical vertebrae, access can be achieved via the anterolateral (between the airways and the carotid sheath), posterolateral (posterior to the carotid sheath), and direct posterior approaches.

Gerald Wyse, H. Hong, and Kieran Murphy

Patients with recurrent head and neck cancer have poor quality of life and suffer dismally from debilitating symptoms. Ablative techniques offer patients an alternative, minimally invasive treatment option. As a palliative treatment, they improve quality of life with decreased pain, improved function and appearance. In addition, there is a reduction in tumor bulk and analgesia requirements. Advantages include a reduction in procedural cost, avoidance of complex repetitive surgeries, and an ability to visualize the treated area at the time of the procedure. Ablation therapies are an evolving and exciting treatment option in the head and neck, but a consensus on appropriate indications is currently unclear.

Classical anatomists have provided detailed description of the arterial collateral pathways found in the head and neck. The small branches building this intricate network are difficult to access. The arterial map inherited from the anatomists has been put to the test with detailed high-resolution vascular imaging. Superselective angiography has helped rediscover the complexity of the craniocervical arterial network. The concept of dangerous collaterals or dangerous anastomoses was born with the advent of endovascular therapy. Although dangerous anastomoses of the skull base are described in the literature, variations and collateral pathways have been overlooked or misunderstood. This article reviews normal orbital arterial vascularization and its principal variations.

Juvenile nasopharyngeal angiofibromas and paragangliomas are the most common hypervascular tumors of the head and neck that require embolization as an adjunct to surgery. A detailed understanding of the functional vascular anatomy of the external carotid artery is necessary for safe and effective endovascular therapy. Embolization, using a transarterial technique and particulate agents, a direct puncture technique and liquid embolic agents, or both techniques may allow for complete devascularization of hypervascular tumors of the head and neck. Effective embolization of these tumors results in a significant reduction of blood loss during surgery and allows for complete resection of the tumors. Use of meticulous technique and a thorough knowledge of functional anatomy of the head and neck vasculature are essential.

Mulliken and Glowacki's seminal classification of vascular anomalies into vascular tumors (with infantile hemangiomas being paradigmatic) versus nontumorous vascular malformations has been as important in the head and neck region as elsewhere. These latter are congenital, have an equal gender incidence, virtually always grow in size with the patient during childhood, and virtually never involute spontaneously. The vascular malformations can in turn be subclassified into high-flow and low-flow. Our focus is on the low-flow malformations, which include those with venous, lymphatic, and, to a lesser extent, capillary components. We address diagnostic and clinical characteristics, particularly insofar as they relate to the structures of the head and neck, and discuss neurointerventional management in some detail.

Head and neck high-flow vascular malformations are uncommon lesions whose management presents a clinical challenge. Although in some rare cases a complete cure is possible, in the vast majority the primary objective is symptom control, cosmesis improvement, and preservation of vital functions. Striving for "complete" treatment in most cases results in potentially devastating clinical and cosmetic outcome. Collateral supply via intracranial vessels is not uncommon, and scrupulous efforts to avoid complications related to inadvertent intracranial embolization or venous thrombosis are mandatory. Regardless of therapeutic goal, close long-term follow-up for lesion recurrence is necessary. Recent demonstration of syndromic associations for some subsets of HFVMs holds out the promise of the future development of medical therapy for these difficult lesions.

Carotid cavernous fistulas (CCFs) are abnormal communications between the carotid arterial system and the cavernous sinus. CCFs are broadly classified as either direct or indirect. Surgical treatment of CCFs is technically difficult and is associated with significant morbidity. Endovascular techniques from either an arterial or a venous approach have become the mainstay of treatment given the recent advances in endovascular technology. This article provides an overview of various endovascular approaches available for the treatment of CCFs.

Cervical arterial dissections and dissecting aneurysms are relatively rare pathologies, but can be associated with significant morbidity from ischemic complications. We review the challenges in diagnosing cervical arterial dissections, their unique clinical presentations and imaging characteristics. Although the majority of cervical dissections heal spontaneously with medical management, we discuss the specific indications for surgical or endovascular treatment to prevent thromboembolic complications. Furthermore, we provide a detailed technical review on endovascular stent reconstruction, the primary interventional option for symptomatic cervical dissections and dissecting aneurysms refractory to medical management.

Carotid blowout syndrome can be a life-threatening late complication of surgical and radiation therapy for head and neck tumors in the vicinity of the cervical carotid artery. The syndrome spans a spectrum of pathology from impending to acute rupture of the artery. These cases are uncommon, can be dramatic in terms of blood loss, and are often true emergencies. The optimal management of these patients requires quick recognition, and often advanced trauma life-support skills and creative endovascular solutions. Definitive endovascular treatment is the therapy of choice in this condition; open surgical options are very limited. In this article, we present some background information regarding the clinical and pathologic aspects of the syndrome and our experience in endovascular management.

Foreword

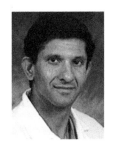

Suresh K. Mukherji, MD
Consulting Editor

There has been an increasingly steady growth in the interest of minimally invasive interventional procedures in the head and neck. Endovascular approach has been the mainstay for interventions in the head and neck, especially in the management of head and neck bleeding, pre-operative embolization of vascular tumors and intra-arterial targeted chemotherapy for malignant neoplasms. Endovascular techniques have replaced surgery as the procedure of choice in the treatment of carotid blowout syndrome and carotid cavernous fistulas. There have been recent numerous advancements in direct percutaneous approaches for a variety of head and neck interventions. Image-guided biopsy allows access to nearly every space in the supra-hyoid and the infra-hyoid neck and has nearly replaced open surgical procedures for tissue sampling. Tissue ablation techniques are emerging as minimally invasive alternatives in the treatment of advanced head and neck tumors.

In this issue, Dr. Dheeraj Gandhi has assembled a group of gifted authors to provide a comprehensive update on interventional procedures of the head and neck. This is a very unique collection of articles, with topics that include interventional management of vascular malformations, updates on various percutaneous ablative procedures, and endovascular management of a variety of head and neck vascular abnormalities, including carotid blowout, carotidocavernous fistula, and vascular tumors.

As many of you may know, Dr. Gandhi and I were colleagues at the University of Michigan for many years. I consider him a very close, personal friend and one of the most talented neurointerventionalists that I have ever had the privilege with whom to work. I am delighted that he accepted our invitation on this unique and singularly challenging topic of interventional head and neck imaging.

Suresh K. Mukherji, MD
Neuroradiology and Head and Neck Radiology
Radiology, Otolaryngology Head Neck Surgery
and Radiation Oncology
University of Michigan Health System
1500 E. Medical Center Drive
Ann Arbor, MI 48109-0030, USA

E-mail address:
mukherji@med.umich.edu (S.K. Mukherji)

doi:10.1016/j.nic.2009.03.002
1052-5149/09/$ – see front matter

neuroimaging.theclinics.com

Preface

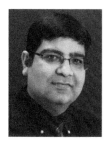

Dheeraj Gandhi, MD
Guest Editor

Minimally invasive, interventional techniques are rapidly evolving and finding an increasing number of applications in the head and neck. Much of this evolution has been technologically driven, particularly as a result of advances in high-resolution imaging techniques, catheter and guide-wire technology, newer embolic agents, and vascular reconstruction devices. These new techniques and devices allow unsurpassed distal vascular access, careful real-time monitoring, and, most importantly, safer performance of complex procedures.

Endovascular and percutaneous interventions in the head and neck region require not only a detailed understanding of complex cross-sectional and vascular anatomy, but also functional anatomy of the extra-cranial and intra-cranial vascular territories, knowledge of potentially dangerous anastomoses, and familiarity with contemporary neuroimaging techniques.

For many years, endovascular approach has been the mainstay for interventions in the head and neck, especially in the management of head and neck bleeding, pre-operative embolization of vascular tumors, and intra-arterial targeted chemotherapy for malignant neoplasms. Endovascular techniques have replaced surgery as the procedure of choice in the treatment of carotid blowout syndrome and carotid cavernous fistulas. In selected instances, endovascular reconstruction can play a useful role in the management of cervical dissections and traumatic vascular injuries.

In recent years, there has been a steadily increasing interest in direct percutaneous approach for a variety of head and neck interventions. Image-guided needle biopsy allows access to nearly every space in the supra-hyoid and the infra-hyoid neck and has nearly replaced open surgical procedures for tissue sampling. Tissue ablation techniques are emerging as minimally invasive alternatives in the treatment of advanced head and neck tumors. These techniques are still in their infancy as far as head and neck lesions are concerned but are likely an important area of potential growth.

Percutaneous techniques are now being increasingly utilized in the embolization of vascular malformations as well as hyper-vascular tumors of the head and neck. These methods permit an easy and direct access to the vascular bed that is not hampered by small size of the arterial feeders, proximal steno-occlusive arterial disease, or vascular tortuosity. With percutaneous approach, there is a potential to achieve more complete devascularization with possibly reduced risk of complications.

This issue of *Neuroimaging Clinics of North America* captures many facets of intervention in the head and neck. Although it is impossible to cover all aspects of interventional neuroradiology of head and neck in a single issue, an emphasis has been placed on providing an update on the current state of the art, discussion of recently introduced techniques and materials, and a glimpse into areas of future growth.

I would like to express my sincere appreciation and thanks to all the authors for their hard work, insight, and attention to detail. The authors share a genuine interest and passion for head and neck interventions, and this fact is reflected in their excellent contributions. My hope is that the readers will enjoy this issue and find the articles stimulating and useful in their daily practice.

I am grateful to Dr. Suresh Mukherji for extending a kind invitation for me to serve as guest editor.

neuroimaging.theclinics.com

It has been a privilege and honor for me to participate in this prestigious journal. I would like to acknowledge the support of Ms. Lydia Gregg for generously contributing through her wonderful medical illustrations for this issue, including the one on the cover.

Lastly, I wish to thank Mr. Donald Mumford, senior developmental editor, and Ms. Lisa Richman, editor, and their staff at Elsevier for their support, professionalism, and assistance in the publication of this issue.

For my wife Bobby, a true friend and love of my life: thank you for your endless support and friendship.

For my beautiful and adorable daughters Shreya and Diya: thank you for your hugs, smiles, and kisses.

For my parents: thank you for your encouragement at every step of my way.

Dheeraj Gandhi, MD
Johns Hopkins University and Hospitals
Departments of Radiology, Neurology,
and Neurosurgery
Division of Interventional Neuroradiology
600 N Wolfe St/Radiology B-100
Baltimore, MD 21287

E-mail address:
dgandhi2@jhmi.edu (D. Gandhi)

State of the Art Head and Neck Imaging for the Endovascular Specialist

Dheeraj Gandhi, MD[a,b,*], Sudhir Kathuria, MD[a],
Sameer A. Ansari, MD, PhD[c], Gaurang Shah, MD[d],
Joseph J. Gemmete, MD[d]

KEYWORDS

- CT angiography • MR angiography • Perfusion imaging
- Head neck imaging • Interventional nueroradiology

Image-guided interventions have undergone a rapid evolution in the last two decades. As compared with open surgical procedures, image-guided techniques offer minimally invasive diagnostic and therapeutic alternatives for various vascular and nonvascular head and neck pathologies. Recent advances in noninvasive imaging not only provide faster and dynamic images but also greater anatomic coverage and improved resolution. Physiologic imaging techniques, such as tissue perfusion, spectroscopy, and thermal mapping, are finding increased use in the management of various head and neck disorders.

Head and neck interventions can be performed by percutaneous, endovascular, or a combination of these approaches. Percutaneous procedures include biopsies, aspirations, sclerotherapy, and newer radiofrequency and cryoablation techniques. Transarterial endovascular approach forms the mainstay of treatment for head and neck bleeding, as well as intra-arterial targeted chemotherapy of neoplasms. Combined percutaneous and endovascular approaches can be useful in the treatment of craniofacial vascular malformations and highly vascular tumors.[1]

Cross-sectional imaging modalities including CT, CT angiography (CTA), MR imaging, MR angiography (MRA), and positron emission tomography (PET) have become an integral part of initial work-up of various head and neck disorders. CT and MR imaging can also provide image guidance during the percutaneous procedures. Latest multidetector CT (MDCT) scanners allow the imaging of larger volumes at much faster speed while maintaining excellent resolution and image quality. CT fluoroscopy and various hybrid imaging systems are tremendous assets in performing various head and neck procedures with greater safety and accuracy. Recently introduced dynamic CTA and four-dimensional MRA techniques can provide hemodynamic information of both the arterial and venous systems in the head and neck. These techniques are helpful in noninvasive evaluation of vascular abnormalities, such as arteriovenous malformations, arteriovenous fistulae, steno-occlusive lesions, and hypervascular masses.

[a] Division of Interventional Neuroradiology, Department of Radiology, Johns Hopkins University and Hospitals, 600 North Wolfe Street, Radiology B-100, Baltimore, MD 21287, USA
[b] Department of Neurosurgery, Johns Hopkins University and Hospitals, 600 North Wolfe Street, Radiology B-100, Baltimore, MD 21287, USA
[c] Johns Hopkins University and Hospitals, Departments of Radiology, Neurology, and Neurosurgery, Division of Interventional Neuroradiology, 600 N Wolfe St/Radiology B-100, Baltimore, MD 21287, USA
[d] Department of Radiology, University of Michigan Health System, 1500 E. Medical Center Drive, BID 330, Ann Arbor, MI 48109, USA
* Corresponding author. Division of Interventional Neuroradiology, Department of Radiology, Johns Hopkins University and Hospitals, 600 North Wolfe Street, Radiology B-100, Baltimore, MD 21287.
E-mail address: dgandhi2@jhmi.edu (D. Gandhi).

Neuroimag Clin N Am 19 (2009) 133–147
doi:10.1016/j.nic.2009.02.002

The role of perfusion imaging is expected to grow in the management of head and neck vascular pathologies (**Fig. 1**). Perfusion imaging, whether performed with CT or MR imaging, evaluates dynamic microscopic blood flow changes through a region of interest. Changes in tissue signal intensity (MR imaging) or attenuation (CT) are measured during a dynamic contrast infusion. Recent literature suggests that perfusion techniques could play an important role in determining which patients with head and neck carcinomas would benefit from medical treatment as opposed to surgical treatment.[2] New developments in thermal imaging are helping to optimize thermal ablations by providing better control at the tumor margins. Continuously evolving imaging techniques play an increasingly important role in the overall care of patients with various head and

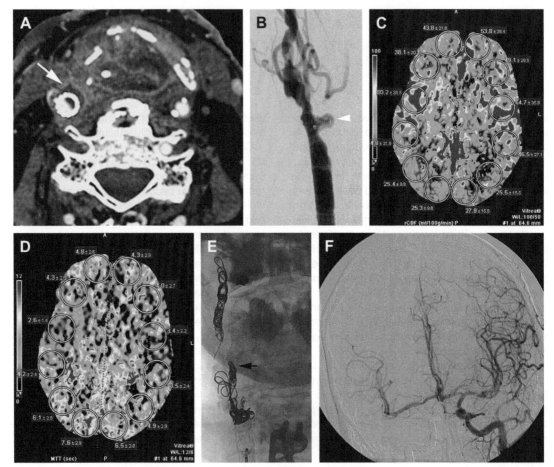

Fig. 1. A 65-year-old patient with previously treated supraglottic laryngeal carcinoma presented with profuse hemoptysis. A pseudoaneurysm arising from the distal right common carotid artery was treated with a stent graft (not shown). The patient presented 11 weeks later with another episode of profuse hemorrhage from his tracheostomy site. (*A*) Neck CTA shows a rim-enhancing fluid collection (*arrow*) adjacent to the stent graft in the right common carotid artery (CCA) indicating infection. (*B*) Common carotid angiogram at this time reveals a recurrent carotid blowout (*arrowhead*) at the distal end of the stent graft. (*C, D*) Given the profuse bleeding, a carotid sacrifice was considered. An awake clinical temporary balloon test occlusion before permanent sacrifice was not an option because the patient was intubated and unable to co-operate with this study. A temporary balloon occlusion of right internal carotid artery with simultaneous CT perfusion of the brain was performed to assess the adequacy of circle of Willis. Images of cerebral blood flow (*C*) and mean transit time (*D*) with balloon inflated in the right internal carotid artery show symmetric flow and mean transit times in bilateral hemispheres suggesting presence of adequate collateral network. (*E*) The internal carotid artery and external carotid artery (*arrow*) were occluded with coils and the common carotid artery was sacrificed proximal to the pseudoaneurysm. (*F*) An angiogram of the left common carotid artery after the right common carotid artery sacrifice demonstrates robust flow in the right anterior circulation by a patent anterior communicating artery. (*From* Gandhi D, et al. Interventional neuroradiology of head and neck. Am J Neuroradiol 2008;29:1806–15; with permission.)

neck disorders and assist the interventional neuro-radiologist in performing safer and effective interventions in the head and neck.

CT

The advent of CT in the late 1970s enabled direct visualization of the soft tissues and its pathology for the first time because of its high contrast resolution.[3] With further development, spiral CT scanners offered faster imaging algorithms and the possibility to image entire anatomic regions relatively quickly. Introduction of slip-ring technology allows the scanner gantry to rotate continuously with concurrent patient table movement. At that speed, most patients are able to hold their breath for the entire imaging session. This improves image quality by eliminating artifacts related to patient motion and breathing. The continuous image acquisition without gaps between slices obtained through helical scanning provides volumetric data that can be reconstructed to produce three-dimensional images. Displaying the entire volume of organs and vessels increases the likelihood of detecting very small lesions.[4]

MDCT systems have been a revolutionary advancement in CT technology. They provide greater anatomic coverage, higher spatial resolution, faster acquisition times, and improved image quality. These faster scanning techniques improve temporal resolution, resulting in dynamic images of the arterial and venous systems. The ability to obtain isotropic volumetric data with superior spatial resolution enables high-quality three-dimensional picture displays of the curved vascular structures. This is specifically advantageous in evaluation of head and neck vascular pathologies, such as atherosclerosis, dissections, traumatic injury, and pseudoaneurysms. Today's state-of-the-art postprocessing software helps delineate pathology with multiplanar imaging, and gathers important information for planning challenging endovascular procedures.

MDCT technology has witnessed rapid development from 1 row of detectors to 4, 16, and 64 rows followed by dual-source CT scanning. The advent of dual-source CT scanners is a significant shift in the further evolution of CT machines. Designed with two X-ray tubes and two detector arrays, the dual-source scanner can capture data nearly twice as fast as previous scanners.[5] The main difference is that the dual-source CT has two X-ray sources and two 64-slice detector arrays as compared with the previous generation of CT scanners, which had a single X-ray source and single 64-row detector.

Recently, a 320-slice CT scanner with five times greater detector coverage than 64-slice CT scanners has been introduced. Using this new scanner, 16-cm (or 6.3-in) Z-axis coverage is now possible in less than 1 second and just one rotation of its gantry. In comparison, a 64-slice CT scanner images only 1.3 inches at a time, leading to relatively longer scan times. One of the major benefits of this scanner is reduced radiation exposure and contrast dose to the patient. The 320-slice CT scanner is extremely fast, taking just one revolution (0.35 seconds) to scan the entire brain. It also has the capability to scan a region repetitively, providing extremely fast and precise information on the functionality of an organ. For example, comprehensive imaging of patients presenting with acute stroke symptoms can be accomplished within 60 seconds. At The Johns Hopkins Hospital, the stroke protocol on 320-slice scanner provides a noncontrast head CT, dynamic (four-dimensional) CT angiogram of the entire brain, and whole-brain perfusion CT using only 50 mL of contrast and the scanning can be accomplished in less than 1 minute. This information is key to rapid assessment and treatment of acute stroke and other neurovascular disorders.

CT ANGIOGRAPHY

CTA is a rapid, noninvasive imaging technique that can produce high-quality angiographic projections of the cervical and cerebral vasculature after intravenous injection of radiographic contrast media. Although it has been in use since the early 1980s, marked improvements in this technique and postprocessing algorithms have occurred with the advent of helical and multislice CT scanners.

Using commercially available software, one can generate two-dimensional and three-dimensional images of vessels from the raw data. These reconstructed images can be viewed from any angle and with varied window settings. Shaded surface displays and maximum intensity projection are the most popular algorithms. It is also possible to view the inner surface of the vessel wall and navigate along the vessel lumen (intra-arterial endoscopy).[6]

In addition to becoming a first-line imaging tool for the assessment of cervicocranial atherosclerotic disease, the role of CTA is also expanding in the assessment of anatomic variations, vascular injuries, dissections, and head and neck masses.[7,8] CTA not only provides useful information on the vascular anatomy and pathology in the neck, but also helps evaluate the patency of circle of Willis. The information gained from CTA allows the head and neck interventionalist to perform more focused angiographic evaluation, thereby limiting the contrast and radiation dose from complex endovascular procedures. Additionally, CTA of head and neck can be easily combined with CT perfusion of the brain. This combined CTA–CT perfusion survey study provides comprehensive imaging assessment of the vascular pathology and its effect on the brain perfusion (see **Fig. 1**).

CTA is extremely useful in the evaluation of patients with head and neck cancer presenting with acute hemorrhage.[9] Although digital subtraction angiography (DSA) is often performed in these patients and still considered gold standard, its interpretation can be confusing. In such patients, often with advanced head and neck carcinomas, postsurgical or postradiation changes commonly result in luminal irregularities or deformities in multiple arterial vessels making it difficult to pinpoint the exact source of hemorrhage. CTA can offer information that is complementary to DSA. It may provide increased sensitivity in detecting slow-filling pseudoaneurysms because of prolonged injection of contrast versus the rapid and transient injection during DSA (**Fig. 2**). CTA can assess the vessel wall directly and provides information regarding the proximity of arterial structures to tumors or the aerodigestive tract. The authors almost always obtain a CTA in patients with suspected carotid blowouts. The information obtained on CTA helps in localization of the bleeding vessel and endovascular treatment planning (see **Fig. 2**).

Several MDCT scanners now allow acquisition of dynamic scans with a wider scan range and faster acquisition times. Dynamic CTA techniques can provide both morphologic and blood flow hemodynamic information of various vascular lesions. In cases of complex arteriovenous malformations and fistulas, dynamic CTA allows identification of feeding arteries, nidus, and draining vessels and enhances the preoperative anatomic assessment of such vascular lesions (**Fig. 3**).[10]

CT FLUOROSCOPY

Deep-seated head and neck lesions have traditionally been evaluated by surgical exploration. The anatomic complexity of various structures including the vessels, airway, nerves, and bones demands a high level of imaging accuracy. CT with its high spatial and contrast resolution provides excellent delineation of these intervening structures and enables planning for safe percutaneous access to the target lesions. CT fluoroscopy involves a display of continuously updated images produced by continuous rotation of the CT tube. The operator at the bedside can typically control

the couch position. CT fluoroscopy is performed at similar kilovolt but much lower milliampere settings compared with conventional CT scanning. It combines the benefits of conventional CT with the added value of a real-time imaging capability.

The CT fluoroscopy system requirements include a slip ring technology for continuous rotation, parallel processing hardware, and high heat capacity. Although continuous scanning modes are available and offer the capability for real-time imaging, most head and neck procedures can be safely performed with intermittent, short bursts of fluoroscopy to adjust the position of an advancing needle. Carlson and colleagues[11] showed that the patient absorbed dose is 94% lower with CT fluoroscopy than with conventional CT. This was accomplished by using an intermittent technique and selecting low fluoroscopic parameters.

CT-guided fluoroscopy greatly alleviates the tedious needle manipulation under traditional CT guidance and significantly shortens CT-guided procedures. CT-guided biopsies and abscess drainages are safely performed percutaneously with equal efficacy using small needles and catheters instead of large surgical incisions.[12] Several types of nerve blocks and radiofrequency nerve ablation procedures including the trigeminal and mandibular nerves can also be performed with safety and with accuracy.[4,13–15] CT fluoroscopy is extremely helpful in approaching difficult areas of the head and neck, including the parapharyngeal, prevertebral, and carotid spaces and pathology involving the skull base and cervical spine (**Fig. 4**).

MR IMAGING AND MR ANGIOGRAPHY

MR imaging techniques play a significant role in assisting and planning diagnostic and therapeutic procedures performed in the head and neck region. Besides providing excellent soft tissue detail and information on vessel morphology, it can provide measurements of blood perfusion and flow. MR perfusion imaging can assist in the clinical decision-making process, such as whether an important blood vessel like internal carotid artery can be safely sacrificed to avoid devastating complications of carotid blowout or severe traumatic injury. Evaluation of low-flow vascular malformations in the head and neck (venous, lymphatic, and capillary malformations) is best performed with MR imaging. Optimal MR imaging studies include fat-saturated T1-weighted sequences before and after gadolinium, fat-saturated T2-weighted or inversion recovery sequences, gradient echo-weighted sequences, and dynamic MR imaging with gadolinium to

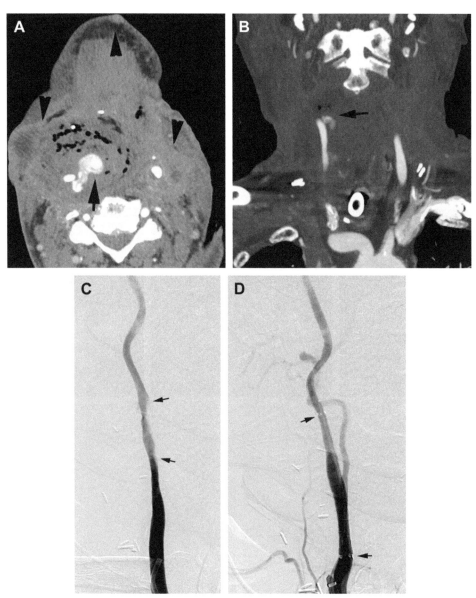

Fig. 2. A 75-year-old man with previous history of pharyngectomy, laryngectomy, bilateral neck dissection, and chemoradiation therapy for glottic carcinoma presented with pulsatile bleeding from his neck. (A) Axial source image of CTA reveals extensive recurrent mass and metastases bilaterally in the neck (*arrowheads*) with encasement of bilateral carotid arteries. Additionally, there is air in the tumor in the right neck suggesting a fistulous connection with the neopharynx. There is frank extravasation of contrast from the right common carotid artery (*arrow*) consistent with blowout of the right carotid artery. (B) Coronal CTA of the same patient reveals the site of extravasation (*arrow*) from the right CCA. The patient was emergently taken to the angiography laboratory. (C) Anteroposterior view of right CCA angiogram reveals narrowing and irregularity of the right CCA suggestive of tumor extension and infiltration (*arrows*). Note that the angiography fails to delineate the active contrast extravasation. As in this patient, CTA often provides a complementary assessment to DSA and helps in planning and targeting the appropriate vessels for endovascular therapy. (D) A covered stent (*arrows*) was placed in the right common carotid artery. This was used as a temporizing measure because the patient had a very limited life expectancy. The covered stent was successful in preventing further episodes of bleeding in this patient.

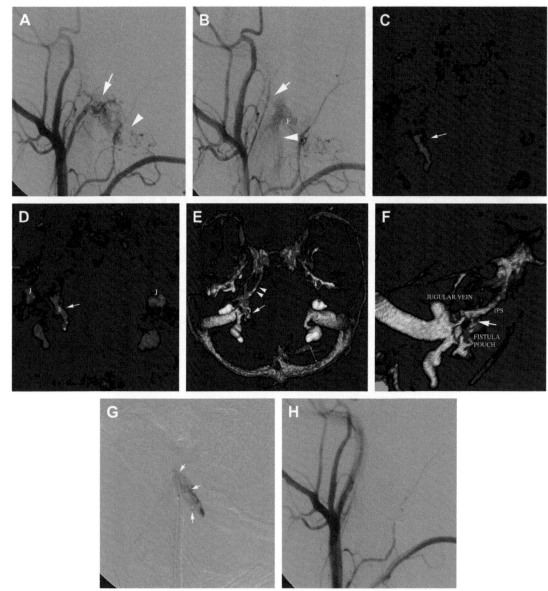

Fig. 3. Use of dynamic CT angiography/venography in planning treatment of a skull base fistula. A 52-year-old woman presented with disabling tinnitus in her right ear. Routine MRI was unremarkable and she underwent an angiogram for further evaluation. (*A*) Lateral views of the right external carotid artery reveal a skull base dural arteriovenous fistula. The fistula is supplied by ascending pharyngeal artery (*arrow*) and mastoid branch of the occipital artery (*arrowhead*). (*B*) An image in slightly later phase demonstrates the fistulous pouch (F) and some filling of the inferior petrosal sinus (*arrow*) and the jugular vein (*arrowhead*). (*C–E*) A dynamic CT venogram on 320-slice CT shows early appearance of the fistulous pouch (*arrow*) in image C and later opacification of jugular veins (J) and the inferior petrosal sinus (*arrowhead*). The source images localized this fistula to the right hypoglossal canal (dural fistula of anterior condylar vein or hypoglossal venous plexus). (*F*) A focused, magnified view of later phase of CT venogram reveals the connection (*arrow*) between the fistula pouch (F) and the inferior petrosal sinus (IPS). (*G*) With the knowledge and understanding of this anatomy, the fistula pouch could be easily catheterized for embolization. Arrows denote the course of the microcatheter from IPS into the venous pouch. (*H*) The venous pouch of the fistula was occluded with platinum coils. A control angiogram in the lateral projection reveals complete occlusion of the fistula.

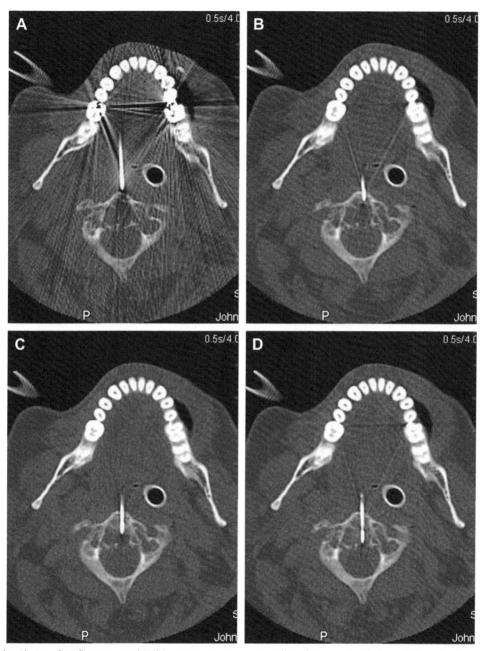

Fig. 4. (A–D) Use of CT fluoroscopy (CTF) in percutaneous approach to deep cervical lesions. This patient presented with neck pain and solitary lytic lesion involving the C2 vertebral body. Transoral biopsy of C2 vertebra under general anesthesia was planned. Successive images using CTF demonstrate transoral placement of vertebral biopsy needle. The tissue sample revealed plasmacytoma. The needle path and the depth of the needles can be exquisitely monitored with CTF technique. Using CTF, the procedure times are significantly shortened, interventions can be performed accurately, and the operator can stay with the patient throughout the procedure.

assess the dynamics of contrast uptake within these lesions.

Head and neck imaging requires high-resolution scanning to delineate small anatomic and pathologic structures. Higher field strength magnets (most commonly 3 T) have a clear advantage over 1.5-T systems, providing higher signal-to-noise ratio and improved spatial and temporal resolution.[16] High spatial resolution, heavily T2-weighted images can be generated using balanced steady-state gradient echo imaging techniques, such as "constructive interference in the steady-state" and "fast imaging employing steady-state acquisition with phase cycling." These techniques provide near isotropic voxels and the capability to reconstruct images in any desired plane. Exquisite detail of fluid-containing structures can be achieved at the expense of decreased tissue contrast. This characteristic makes it particularly suitable for imaging the labyrinth, cochlea, internal auditory canals, and cranial nerves or vessels within the subarachnoid cisterns. Diffusion-weighted imaging is useful in the evaluation of certain head and neck malignancies and apparent diffusion coefficient measurements may be useful specifically to characterize these lesions. A significant difference between apparent diffusion coefficient values has been found between benign and malignant lesions of the sinonasal region, parotid gland, and skull base.[17]

MR imaging and MRA play a complementary role in the assessment of vascular pathologies, such as cervical arterial dissections. A combination of MR imaging and MRA studies is generally considered the primary investigation in patients with suspected dissections. MR imaging is capable of demonstrating a typical evolution of signal intensity related to the paramagnetic effects of the products of hemoglobin breakdown in the vessel wall. In the early and chronic stage, the hematoma usually demonstrates isointense signal to the surrounding structures, whereas between 1 and 8 weeks, it is almost invariably bright on T1-weighted images.[18] Addition of MRA imaging improves the detection of stenosis, occlusion, and dissecting aneurysms. Sensitivity and specificity figures in excess of 90% have been reported for carotid dissection using a combination of MR imaging and MRA techniques. Of note, MR imaging with MRA is less sensitive and specific in the diagnosis of vertebral artery dissections.[18]

High-resolution MR imaging is one of the most promising modalities available today for visualizing the carotid atherosclerotic plaque, characterizing its morphology and tissue composition (Fig. 5). This technique is also capable of studying atherosclerosis progression or treatment-induced regression.[19] Imaging is now evolving from the mere detection of luminal narrowing and plaque morphology to identifying cellular and molecular processes occurring within the plaque. Fibrocellular tissue within the atheroma can be detected from its selective enhancement after administration of a gadolinium-based contrast agent.[20] Some of these novel techniques, such as ultrasmall particles of iron oxide–enhanced MR imaging to detect macrophage activity,[21] fluorodeoxyglucose PET to image metabolic activity and inflammation within the atherosclerotic

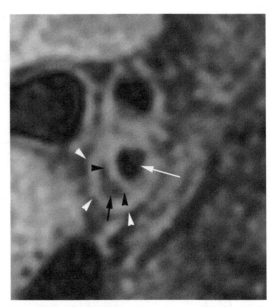

Fig. 5. MR imaging of atheromatous plaque. High-resolution T1-weighted black blood MR image acquired on a 1.5-T scanner demonstrating an asymptomatic plaque (*white arrowheads*) of the right internal carotid artery with a fibrous cap (*black arrowheads*) separating the lumen (*white arrow*) from the lipid core (*black arrow*). (*Courtesy of* Bruce Wasserman, MD, Baltimore, MD.)

plaque,[22] and radiolabelled Annexin V in detecting apoptosis[23] have already been used in human patients with promising results.[24] This combination of structural and molecular imaging techniques will soon revolutionize the way patients with carotid atherosclerosis are diagnosed and managed.

Catheter angiography with digital subtraction still remains the gold standard for the evaluation and characterization of the cervical and cranial vasculature. However, safer alternatives are being developed because of a very small risk of stroke from arterial catheterizations, risk of ionizing radiation, and higher cost of endovascular procedures. Recently, MRA has emerged as a competitive modality for the evaluation of arterial and venous anatomy in the head and neck. Several new improved techniques and sequences are being developed at a rapid pace. Traditional flow-sensitive techniques, such as time-of-flight MRA, lack temporal resolution and are limited by flow-related artifacts and low spatial resolution. Contrast-enhanced MRA overcomes many limitations of time-of-flight MRA and produces high-resolution three-dimensional volume acquisition. However, it provides no dynamic information and is dependent on accurate timing for optimal visualization of the arterial tree. Routine three-dimensional contrast-enhanced technique reduces some of the flow-related artifacts, but is unable to provide temporal resolution necessary in the evaluation of complex vascular lesions.[25] Time-resolved MRA has overcome many of these challenges and has particular advantages for imaging vascular malformations because it provides hemo-dynamic information and anatomic asses-ssment.[26] In addition, the recent development of parallel imaging allows further reduction of acqui-sition time providing improved temporal resolution while maintaining high spatial resolution. Multiple data sets are obtained with parallel imaging to reduce the scan time, taking advantage of many integrated panoramic coils. The individual data sets are then combined to generate the final image.[27] Combining time-resolved MRA with parallel imaging can produce good quality images using smaller contrast volumes. Various modifica-tions of subsampling k-space are being devel-oped, such as one with exclusion of the corners of k-space that can significantly reduce the scan time, and are being used with parallel imaging.

By providing relative flow quantification in the feeding arteries, and detailed characterization of complex, dynamic blood flow patterns, the four-dimensional flow technique can supplement both current noninvasive and invasive imaging of intra-cranial and extracranial vascular disorders.[28] Four-dimensional dynamic MRA is an effective means to evaluate multidirectional blood flow within vessels. It uses various techniques that accelerate ultrafast gradient echo sequences, such as parallel acquisition (SENSE, GRAPPA) and implement segmented readout of k-space with variable refreshment at each phase (TRICKS: time-resolved imaging of contrast kinetics; contrast-enhanced timing angiography; TREAT: time-resolved echo-shared angiographic tech-nique). Combining these techniques can produce sequences with reduced acquisition times, improved temporal resolution, and thereby dynamic imaging (4D-TRAK: four-dimensional time-resolved angiography using keyhole, TRICKS, and TWIST). Time-resolved imaging of contrast kinetics uses extremely rapid acquisition to provide dynamic images of intravascular contrast flow. These methods provide relatively high spatial resolution and dynamic flow informa-tion that has not been previously available without invasive catheter angiography (Fig. 6). The specific advantages of four-dimensional MRA over other modalities include its noninvasive nature, lack of ionizing radiation, better safety profile, and dynamic blood flow assessment. It has been shown to provide critical information in orbital vascular lesions improving the evaluation and management of these patients.[29]

INTERVENTIONAL MR IMAGING

MR imaging–guided interventional procedures involving both bone and soft tissues can be safely and effectively performed in clinical practice. Although CT fluoroscopy currently is the modality of choice for many interventional procedures, MR imaging guidance provides distinct advantages in certain situations. Cysts are often better visualized on MR imaging compared with CT and have been successfully treated under MR imaging guid-ance.[30] Certain bony lesions, such as hemangi-omas, can be very difficult to identify on CT, but are easily detected on MR imaging. A major advantage of MR imaging–guided interventions is lack of radiation exposure to both physicians and patients, especially important in pediatric popula-tion and pregnant patients.

MR imaging–guided cryotherapy for head and neck lesions is advantageous compared with CT-guided cryotherapy. Although CT attenuation of frozen tissue is lower than that of the surrounding soft tissue, the difference in attenuation is small compared with the difference in signal intensity of frozen and unfrozen tissue. MR imaging–guided cryoablation can be performed in multiple planes in real time, does not involve the use of ionizing radiation, and distinctly depicts both ice ball and tumor. Tumors typically have increased signal intensity on T2-weighted images, whereas ice balls cause a signal void. On CT, both tumor and ice ball are hypodense and often cannot be differentiated.[31,32]

Current limitations of interventional MR imaging include longer procedure times, higher cost, and limited availability of instruments. However, devel-opment of new guidance methods and devices is under progress, including faster image acquisition using stronger radiofrequency pulses, increased homogeneity from high field strength magnets, and larger working spaces with shorter bores. These further advancements hold great promise for MR imaging–guided interventions in the near future.

DIGITAL SUBTRACTION ANGIOGRAPHY

DSA of cerebral and head and neck vasculature has been extremely valuable in the diagnosis and evaluation of various vascular lesions, such as aneurysms, arteriovenous malformations, fistulas, and steno-occlusive diseases. It has maintained an essential role in the evaluation and treatment of these disease processes. However, catheter angiography remains an invasive procedure and requires significant experience to perform it safely. In recent years, advances in CTA and MRA

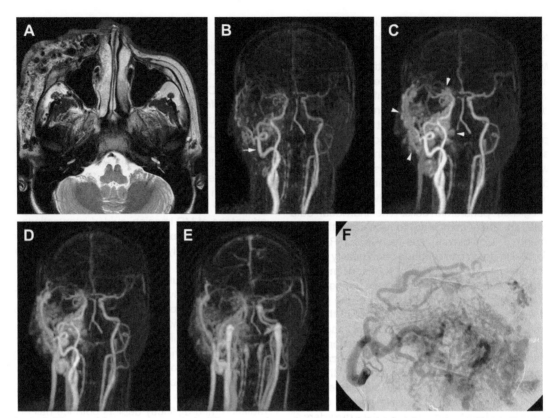

Fig. 6. A 28-year-old woman presented with progressive enlargement of right facial vascular malformation and frequent episodes of bleeding. MR imaging, dynamic MRA, and DSA identified an extremely high-flow, extensive arteriovenous malformation (AVM) of entire right face, periorbital region, and nose. This AVM was deemed inoperable previously and the patient was brought to the authors' center. (*A*) An axial T2-weighted image at the initial presentation reveals extensive AVM. Note the soft tissue enlargement and multiple flow voids in the right face. (*B–E*) Four-dimensional time-resolved angiography using keyhole dynamic MRA images in the coronal plane reveal sequential changes of contrast kinetics in this AVM. The contrast inflow is noted in image *B*. Note that the right external carotid artery (ECA) is hypertrophied (*arrow*) and fills earlier than the left ECA. There is sequential opacification of a large nidus (*arrowheads*) and large draining veins on images *C*, *D*, and *E*. (*F*) Right external carotid angiogram, lateral view DSA reveals markedly hypertrophied branches (superficial temporal, internal maxillary) of right external carotid artery supplying an extensive nidus. (*G*) The patient was treated with staged embolization. This image reveals the extent of the embolic cast in the right face. (*H–K*) Follow-up four-dimensional time-resolved angiography using keyhole MRA on 3-T system (compare with *B–E*) reveals marked devascularization of the AVM. Note the lack of filling of the nidus and decreased size of the right ECA and its branches. Also, note the decreased size of draining veins of the right face and neck (*J, K*). (*L*) Lateral view of the right CCA reveals near complete obliteration of the facial nidus (note the subtraction artifact caused by embolic cast, *arrows*). The only residual vascularity was in the region of medial canthus supplied by hypertrophied ophthalmic artery (*arrowheads*). The patient underwent uncomplicated resection of this AVM with minimal blood loss and is currently undergoing nasal reconstruction.

imaging have replaced DSA in many situations for diagnostic information. However, there are still common situations, such as subarachnoid hemorrhage, where a high negative predictive value for aneurysm with CTA or MRA is not good enough.[33,34]

DSA has also undergone technologic advances with enhanced machine capabilities and new postprocessing software. Current systems are equipped with flat panel detectors and offer significant improvement in low-contrast resolution.

Furthermore, rotational datasets can be used to reconstruct native or contrast CT datasets of the brain, head, and neck. This capability is extremely helpful in neurointerventional procedures. Flatdetector CT has already found its usefulness in stenting for cerebrovascular stenoses, stentassisted aneurysm embolization, and in the management of arteriovenous malformations. Dedicated intracranial stents that are barely visible in plain fluoroscopy can now easily be visualized with high-resolution flat-detector CT. Imaging of

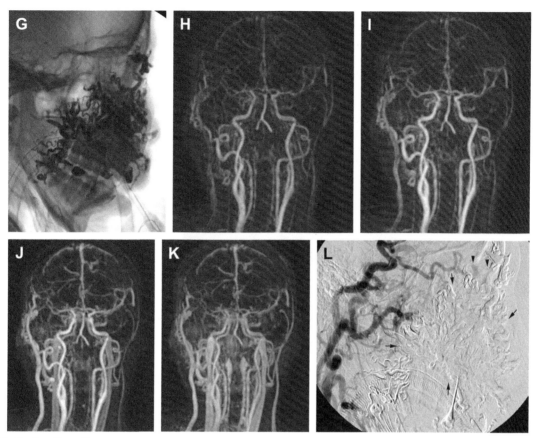

Fig. 6. (continued)

periprocedural hemorrhage, which could previously only be accomplished on conventional CT, is now possible within the angiographic suite with use of flat-detector CT.[35,36] This may help in quick recognition and management of complications during neurointerventional procedures without the need to move the patient to the CT scanner.[36] Although the current descriptions of use of these systems are mostly in reference to intracranial and spinal procedures, this technique will likely gain importance for planning, guiding, and monitoring interventional procedures of the head and neck.

HYBRID IMAGING SYSTEMS

Hybrid PET-CT scanning enables one to find new or recurrent tumors first using metabolism-based PET images and then localizing them accurately with fusion of CT images. This hybrid modality has been found to be superior to the conventional imaging work-up in patients with head and neck malignancies and in the detection of recurrences.[37,38] Additionally, PET-CT may assist in interventional planning of the target lesion for biopsies and reduce the false-negative rate.

X-ray fluoroscopy provides high-resolution real-time (30 frames per second) images using a two-dimensional projection format. It is particularly suited for imaging bones; contrast-enhanced blood flow; and micro devices, such as stents, guidewires, and catheters. MR imaging, however, is excellent for soft tissue and cross-sectional imaging. It provides three-dimensional data sets allowing arbitrary choice of scan planes. Several systems have been developed to combine these two complementary modalities. X-ray fluoroscopy–MR imaging hybrid systems offer excellent temporal and spatial resolution of X-ray and fine soft tissue contrast resolution provided by MR imaging. This is a distinct advantage in procedures involving anesthetized patients with critically positioned needles and interventional instruments and during procedures in which precise image fusion of MR imaging and X-ray images is anticipated.[39]

Another recently developed hybrid system combines CT and DSA technology. In this system, the angiographic suite harbors both DSA equipment and a CT scanner gantry. The authors have had early experience working on a hybrid suite containing single-plane DSA and 64-slice MDCT equipment (DG, SAA, JG). At this time, installation of a biplane DSA suite and 64-slice MDCT is underway at the University of Michigan. Such systems may prove to be ideal for head and neck interventions where percutaneous and endovascular approaches are anticipated (Fig. 7). In the future, a combined biplane DSA-CT system could also be very useful in the treatment of acute stroke. Patients with suspected stroke could be transferred directly from the emergency room to the angiographic suite where CT head, CTA, and CT perfusion could be performed using the CT gantry. If endovascular intervention is indicated, the table could simply be rotated and thrombolysis interventions initiated using the biplane DSA equipment without needing to move or transfer the patient.

Hybrid DSA-CT systems combine the advantages of high spatial and temporal resolution of DSA with the high-contrast, soft tissue resolution obtained by CT. This allows safe placement of endovascular catheters under the angiographic

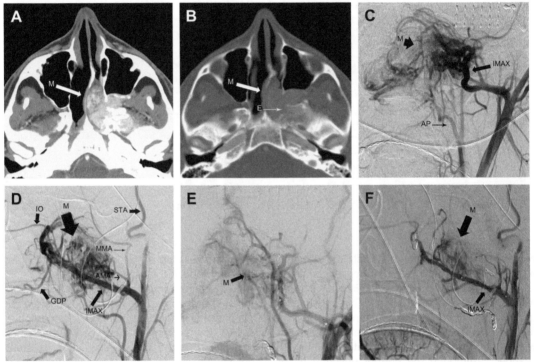

Fig. 7. Embolization of large, hypervascular juvenile nasal angiofibroma using combined endovascular and percutaneous approach. (A) Enhanced CT scan shows a hypervascular mass (M) in the left nasal cavity and the sphenopalatine foramen, suggestive of juvenile nasal angiofibroma. (B) Bone windows demonstrate a large area of erosion (E) of the sphenoid bone and an enlarged sphenopalatine foramen anterior to the area of erosion. Selective anteroposterior (C) and left external carotid (D) angiogram reveals hypertrophied branches of internal maxillary (Imax) and ascending pharyngeal (AP) arteries supplying this mass. AMA, accessory meningeal artery; GDP, greater descending palatine artery; IMAX, internal maxillary artery; IO, infraorbital artery; MMA, middle meningeal artery; STA, superficial temporal artery. (E, F) Transarterial embolization of internal maxillary, accessory pharyngeal, and ascending pharyngeal artery branches feeding this tumor was performed with 300- to 500-μm embospheres and detatchable coils. The anteroposterior (E) and lateral (F) views after the embolization reveal residual tumor blush. Percutaneous needle (N) placement in the mass under CT guidance by infratemporal (G) and transnasal (H) approach is demonstrated. (I) A parenchymogram of the tumor is first performed to ensure correct needle position, to access the distribution of the contrast, and to exclude any retrograde filling of arterial branches or internal carotid artery. M, mass; S, sphenoid sinus; ant, anterior; N, needle. (J) Percutaneous embolization of the tumor with Onyx was subsequently performed. Note the deposition of Onyx (O) cast on this focused lateral view. (K) Postembolization angiogram of left common carotid artery reveals near complete devascularization of the mass. (L) Postprocedure CT scan demonstrates the extent of the Onyx cast (O) on this sagittal view. The patient underwent an uncomplicated resection of this mass with less than 400 mL of blood loss at surgery.

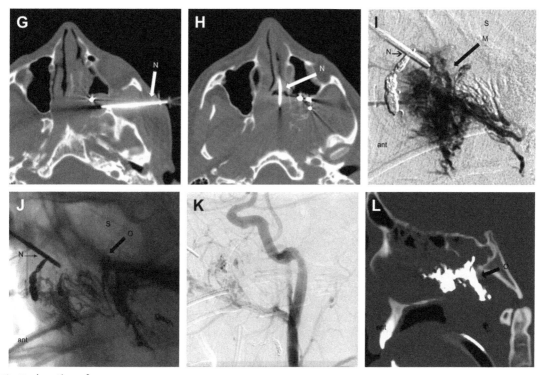

Fig. 7. (*continued*)

system and then switching to the CT gantry to obtain intra-arterial CT angiography. Intra-arterial CTA provides an exceptional level of detail and provides valuable information in the understanding and surgical planning of some complex and small neurovascular pathologic lesions.[40]

SUMMARY

Recent technologic advances including MDCT, dynamic CTA, high-field MR imaging, four-dimensional MRA, and physiologic studies, such as perfusion imaging, have revolutionized the imaging work-up of head, neck, and skull base lesions. These techniques not only provide accurate diagnostic information, but also help plan endovascular therapy. In many instances, these studies provide better evaluation of vascular disease compared with DSA by identifying intramural pathology at an earlier stage. The future holds great promise for interventional neuroradiologists because excellent imaging tools are becoming available that are capable of providing morphologic, hemodynamic, and physiologic information. Furthermore, availability of faster, real-time guidance systems and hybrid systems improves their ability to perform procedures not only in a rapid and safe manner but also with great precision.

REFERENCES

1. Gandhi D, Gemmete JJ, Ansari SA, et al. Interventional neuroradiology of the head and neck. AJNR Am J Neuroradiol 2008;29:1806–15.
2. Zima A, Carlos R, Gandhi D, et al. Can pretreatment CT perfusion predict response of advanced squamous cell carcinoma of the upper aerodigestive tract treated with induction chemotherapy? AJNR Am J Neuroradiol 2007;28:328–34.
3. Bakal CW. Advances in imaging technology and the growth of vascular and interventional radiology: a brief history. J Vasc Interv Radiol 2003;14:855–60.
4. Taguchi K, Anno H. High temporal resolution for multi-slice helical computed tomography. Med Phys 2000;27(5):861–72.
5. Flohr TG, McCollough CH, Bruder H, et al. First performance evaluation of a dual-source CT (DSCT) system. Eur Radiol 2006;16:256–68.
6. Gandhi D. Computed tomography and magnetic resonance angiography in cervico-cranial vascular disease. J Neuroophthalmol 2004;24(4):306–14.

7. Lee J, Fernandes R. Neck masses: evaluation and diagnostic approach. Oral Maxillofac Surg Clin North Am 2008;20:321–37.

8. Perkins JA, Sidhu M, Manning SC, et al. Three-dimensional CT angiography imaging of vascular tumors of the head and neck. Int J Pediatr Otorhinolaryngol 2005;69:319–25.

9. Goodman DN, Hoh BL, Rabinov JD, et al. CT angiography before embolization for hemorrhage in head and neck cancer. AJNR Am J Neuroradiol 2003;24:140–2.

10. Matsumoto M, Kodama N, Endo Y, et al. Dynamic 3D-CT angiography. AJNR Am J Neuroradiol 2007;28:299–304.

11. Carlson SK, Bender CE, Oberg AL, et al. Benefits and safety of CT fluoroscopy in interventional radiologic procedures. Radiology 2001;219:5515–20.

12. vanSonnenberg E, Ferrucci JT Jr, Mueller PR, et al. Percutaneous radiographically guided catheter drainage of abdominal abscesses. JAMA 1982;247:190–2.

13. Kanaplot Y, Savas A, Bekar A, et al. Percutaneous controlled radiofrequency trigeminal rhizotomy for the treatment of idiopathic trigeminal neuralgia: 25-year experience with 1600 patients. Neurosurgery 2001;48:524–32.

14. Gusmao S, Oliveira M, Tazinaffo U, et al. Percutaneous trigeminal nerve radiofrequency rhizotomy guided by computerized tomography fluoroscopy: technical note. J Neurosurg 2003;99:785–6.

15. Koizuko S, Saito S, Kubo K, et al. Percutaneous radio-frequency mandibular nerve rhizotomy guided by CT fluoroscopy. AJNR Am J Neuroradiol 2006;27:1647–8.

16. Aygun N, Zinreich SJ. Head and neck imaging at 3T. Magn Reson Imaging Clin N Am 2006;14:89–95.

17. Wang J, Takashima S, Takayama F, et al. Head and neck lesions: characterization with diffusion-weighted echo-planar MR imaging. Radiology 2001;220:621–30.

18. Rodallec MH, Marteau V, Gerber S, et al. Craniocervical arterial dissection: spectrum of imaging findings and differential diagnosis. Radiographics 2008;28:1711–28.

19. Yuan C, Oikawa M, Miller Z, et al. MRI of carotid atherosclerosis. J Nucl Cardiol 2008;15:266–75.

20. Wasserman BA, Smith WI, Trout HH, et al. Carotid artery atherosclerosis: in vivo morphologic characterization with gadolinium-enhanced double-oblique MR imaging. Initial results. Radiology 2002;223:566–73.

21. Trivedi RA, Mallawarachi C, U-King-Im J, et al. Idenitifying inflamed carotid plaques using in vivo USPIO-enhanced MR imaging to label plaque macrophages. Arterioscler Thromb Vasc Biol 2006;26:1601–6.

22. Tawakol A, Migrino RQ, Bashian GG, et al. In vivo 18F-fluorodeoxyglucose positron emission tomography imaging provides a non-invasive measure of carotid plaque inflammation in patients. J Am Coll Cardiol 2006;48:1818–24.

23. Hartung D, Sarai M, Petrov A, et al. Resolution of apoptosis in atherosclerotic plaque by dietary modification and statin therapy. J Nucl Med 2005;46:2051–6.

24. U-King-Im JM, Tang T, Moustafa RR, et al. Imaging the cellular biology of the carotid plaque. Int J Stroke 2007;2:85–96.

25. Farb RI, McGregor C, Kim JK, et al. Intraccranial arteriovenous malformations: real-time, auto triggered elliptic centric-ordered 3D gadolinium-enhanced MR angiography. Initial assessment. Radiology 2001;220:244–51.

26. Wetzel SG, Bilecen D, Lyrer P, et al. Cerebral dural arteriovenous fustulas: detection by dynamic MR projection angiography. AJR Am J Roentgenol 2000;174:1293–5.

27. Gauvrit JY, Law M, Xu J, et al. Time-resolved MR angiography: optimal parallel imaging method. AJNR Am J Neuroradiol 2007;28:835–8.

28. Sandison GA, Loye MP, Rewcastle JC, et al. X-ray CT monitoring of iceball growth and thermal distribution during cryosurgery. Phys Med Biol 1998;43:3309–24.

29. Kahana A, Lucarelli MJ, Grayev AM, et al. Noninvasive dynamic magnetic resonance angiography with time-resolved imaging of contrast kinetics (TRICKS) in the evaluation of orbital vascular lesions. Arch Ophthalmol 2007;125:1635–42.

30. Takahashi S, Morikawa S, Egawa M, et al. Magnetic resonance imaging-guided percutaneous fenestration of a cervical intradural cyst: case report. J Neurosurg 2003;99:313–5.

31. Tuncali K, Morrison PR, Winalski CS, et al. MR imaging-guided percutaneous cryotherapy of soft tissue and bone metastases: initial experience. AJR Am J Roentgenol 2007;189:232–9.

32. Hope MD, Purcell DD, Hope TA, et al. Complete intracranial arterial and venous blood flow evaluation with 4D flow MR imaging. AJNR Am J Neuroradiol 2009;30:362–6.

33. Kallmes DF, Layton K, Marx WF, et al. Death by non-diagnosis: why emergent CT angiography should not be done for patients with subarachnoid hemorrhage. AJNR Am J Neuroradiol 2007;28:1837–8.

34. Kaufman TJ, Kallmes DF. Diagnostic cerebral angiography: archaic and complication-prone or here to stay for another 80 years? AJR Am J Roentgenol 2008;190:1435–7.

35. Kyriakou Y, Richter G, Dorfler A, et al. Neuroradiologic applications with routine C-arm flat panel detector CT: evaluation of patient dose measurements. AJNR Am J Neuroradiol 2008;29:1930–6.

36. Kalender WA, Kyriakou Y. Flat-detector CT (FD-CT). Eur Radiol 2007;1:828–37.

37. Paulus P, Sambon A, Vivegnis D, et al. 18FDG-PET for the assessment of primary head and neck

tumors: clinical, computed tomography, and histopathological correlation in 38 patients. Laryngoscope 1998;108:1578–83.

38. Schmid DT, Stoeckli SJ, Bandhauer F, et al. Impact of positron emission tomography on the initial staging and therapy in locoregional advanced squamous cell carcinoma of the head and neck. Laryngoscope 2003;113:888–91.

39. Ganguly A, Wen Z, Daniel BL, et al. Truly hybrid X-ray/MR imaging: toward a streamlined clinical system. Acad Radiol 2005;12:1167–77.

40. Gandhi D, Pandey A, Ansari SA, et al. Multi-detector row CT angiography with direct intra-arterial contrast injection for the evaluation of neurovascular disease: technique, applications, and initial experience. AJNR Am J Neuroradiol 2009, in press.

Approaches for Percutaneous Needle Placement for Various Head and Neck Procedures

Sanjay Gupta, MD

KEYWORDS
- Head and neck • Biopsy • Percutaneous
- Neck spaces • Image guidance

Image-guided percutaneous needle placement is required for various diagnostic and therapeutic procedures, including biopsies, ablation procedures, and nerve root and ganglion blocks, in the head and neck region.[1-8] A thorough knowledge of the anatomy of this region is essential for planning a safe route of access for needle placement in deep-seated head and neck lesions because major vessels, nerves, the airway, or osseous structures often intervene in the projected needle path. In this article, we review the various approaches that can be used for percutaneous needle placement in the head and neck region, focusing on the relevant anatomy, technical aspects, and the advantages and limitations of each approach.

ANATOMY

For the purpose of this discussion, it is useful to describe the anatomy in terms of various fascial planes and intervening spaces that exist in the head and neck region, and focus on the important osseous, muscular, vascular, and neural structures that are contained within these fascial spaces. The head and neck area can be divided into suprahyoid and infrahyoid regions.[9,10] The important fascial spaces in the suprahyoid region include the parapharyngeal, masticator, parotid, carotid, pharyngeal mucosal, retropharyngeal, and perivertebral spaces. In the infrahyoid neck,

apart from the inferior extensions of the carotid, retropharyngeal, and perivertebral spaces, three other spaces, namely the visceral and the posterior and anterior cervical spaces, can be identified.

The parapharyngeal space is a pyramidal-shaped fat-containing potential space that extends from the hyoid bone inferiorly to the skull base superiorly, and is bordered by the masticator space anteriorly, the deep parotid space laterally, the pharyngeal mucosal space medially, the carotid space posteriorly, and the lateral extension of the retropharyngeal space posteromedially. The major neurovascular structures that traverse this space include the internal maxillary, middle meningeal, and ascending pharyngeal arteries; the pterygoid venous plexus; and branches of the mandibular nerve.

The pharyngeal mucosal space is medial to the parapharyngeal space and is located deep to the buccopharyngeal fascia in the nasopharynx and oropharynx and contains mucosa, lymphoid tissue, minor salivary glands, and pharyngeal constrictor muscles.

The masticator space extends from the mandible up to the skull base, and has two components: the infratemporal fossa below the zygomatic arch and the temporal fossa above it. Spaces that border the masticator space include the buccal space anteriorly, the parotid space posteriorly, and the parapharyngeal space posteromedially. The contents of the masticator space include the medial and

Department of Diagnostic Radiology, The University of Texas M.D. Anderson Cancer Center, 1515 Holcombe Boulevard, Unit 325, Houston, TX 77030, USA
E-mail address: sgupta@mdanderson.org

Neuroimag Clin N Am 19 (2009) 149–160
doi:10.1016/j.nic.2009.01.002

lateral pterygoid, masseter, and temporalis muscles, the ramus and body of the mandible, and the inferior alveolar branch of the mandibular nerve and the inferior alveolar vessels.

The carotid space extends from the skull base to the aortic arch, and contains the common or the internal carotid artery (depending on the level); the internal jugular vein; sympathetic plexus; cranial nerves IX, X, XI, and XII in the nasopharyngeal portion; cranial nerve X in the oropharyngeal portion and infrahyoid neck; and lymph nodes. The parapharyngeal space forms the anterior boundary of the carotid space in the suprahyoid neck.

The parotid space is located lateral to the parapharyngeal space and posterolateral to the masticator space, extending from the level of the external auditory canal down to the angle of the mandible. The posterior belly of the digastric muscle separates the medial portion of the parotid space from the anterolateral aspect of the carotid space. Apart from the parotid gland, the space contains facial nerve, external carotid artery, retromandibular vein, and lymph nodes.

The retropharyngeal space, which contains fat and lymph nodes only, is a midline space located between the pharyngeal constrictor muscle anteriorly and prevertebral muscles posteriorly. This space extends laterally up to the carotid space.

The perivertebral space lies beneath the deep layer of deep cervical fascia and extends from the skull base to the fourth thoracic vertebral level. The prevertebral portion of this space contains the prevertebral muscles, the vertebral artery and vein, the scalene muscles, the brachial plexus, the phrenic nerve, and the vertebral body, transverse process, and pedicle, whereas the paravertebral portion of this space contains the paravertebral muscles and posterior elements of the cervical vertebrae.

The visceral space is bounded by the middle layer of the deep cervical fascia, extends from the hyoid bone to the mediastinum, and contains the thyroid and parathyroid glands, larynx, hypopharynx, esophagus, trachea, recurrent laryngeal nerve, and lymph nodes. The posterior cervical space is located posterior to the carotid space and lateral to the perivertebral space, and contains the spinal accessory nerve and the preaxillary portion of the brachial plexus. The anterior cervical space, which is located lateral to the visceral space and anterior to the carotid space, does not contain any important structure.

IMAGE GUIDANCE

Image guidance is generally required for various percutaneous procedures in the head and neck region in nonpalpable deep-seated head and neck lesions. Superficial neck nodes, thyroid lesions, and parotid gland lesions can be accessed with sonographic guidance.[11–13] However, the lack of an adequate acoustic window because of overlying bony structures such as the maxilla, mandible, mastoid, and the styloid process and the air-containing aerodigestive system preclude the use of sonographic guidance for many deep-seated head and neck lesions. Fluoroscopy is routinely used for guiding vertebroplasty and discography procedures for cervical spine. Although fluoroscopic-guided needle placement has been used for nerve root and ganglion blocks and for biopsy of cervical spine and skull base lesions, inability to visualize the intervening structures increases the risk of complications. CT, with its high spatial and contrast resolution, is the imaging modality of choice for percutaneous needle placement in nonpalpable deep-seated head and neck lesions.[1,3,5,8,14–16] Air-containing spaces and bony structures do not result in significant image degradation, especially with the use of thin-section collimation. CT allows for excellent delineation of intervening vital structures, permitting safe biopsy path planning. Magnetic resonance imaging (MR imaging), because of its high contrast resolution, its multiplanar imaging capacity allowing the use of double oblique approaches, and its ability to visualize vessels without a contrast agent, has also been used for guiding needle placement in head and neck lesions.[4,6,17] However, the limited availability of open-configuration MR imaging systems, high cost, longer acquisition times, and need for MR imaging–compatible needles has prevented more widespread use of MR imaging guidance for these procedures.

COMPLICATIONS

Image-guided percutaneous needle placement for various head and neck procedures is rarely associated with major complications.[1–8] A thorough knowledge of the cross-sectional anatomy of the head and neck region and careful attention to access trajectory planning minimize the chances of injury to major neural and vascular structures. Minor complications including pain, vasovagal reaction, minor infection, and minor bleeding have been reported. Transient recurrent laryngeal nerve damage has been reported. Trauma to the trachea and esophagus can result in mediastinal or surgical emphysema. Injury to the lung and pleura may occur resulting in pneumothorax, which may require chest tube placement. Review of literature revealed one case report of maxillary artery pseudoaneurysm after needle biopsy of the masticator space lesion.[18]

APPROACHES USED FOR PERCUTANEOUS ACCESS IN SUPRAHYOID HEAD AND NECK
Subzygomatic (Infratemporal, Transcondylar, Sigmoid Notch) Approach

The subzygomatic approach is ideally suited for accessing lesions in the masticator space. In addition to lesions in the infrazygomatic portion of the space, lesions in the suprazygomatic portion (temporal fossa) of the masticator space and the skull base can also be accessed with this approach by using a cranial needle angulation. This approach also allows easy access to lesions in the parapharyngeal, pharyngeal mucosal, and retropharyngeal spaces and the prevertebral portion of the perivertebral space. Furthermore, this approach is used for needle placement in the pterygopalatine fossa for neurolysis of the pterygopalatine ganglion for pain management.

The needle is inserted below the zygomatic arch and is advanced through the intercondylar (sigmoid) notch between the coronoid process anteriorly, the mandibular condyle posteriorly, and the superior border of the mandibular ramus inferiorly. The needle can easily be angulated in various directions (anterior, posterior, cranial, or caudal), permitting access to multiple target sites.[2] The needle traverses the masticator and the parapharyngeal spaces for lesions located in the pharyngeal mucosal, retropharyngeal, and prevertebral spaces and skull base lesions (**Fig. 1**). Cranial needle angulation allows the subzygomatic approach to be used for accessing lesions in the skull base and the suprazygomatic portion of the masticator space. A triangulation method can be used to estimate the required needle angle from contiguous axial CT scans obtained from the level of the planned skin entry site to the level of the target lesion. The needle is inserted below the level of the zygomatic arch and advanced cranially and medially; the needle tip position and angulation are checked with intermittent axial CT scans (**Fig. 2**). Alternatively, a change in the degree of neck flexion can bring the target lesion and the skin entry site into the same axial plane, allowing visualization of the entire needle length in a single axial CT image. Tilting the gantry 10 degrees caudally can also be used to facilitate needle placement in skull base lesions. Occasionally, if passage of need through the notch is difficult, having the patient keep his or her mouth open, preferably with a bite block, can help open up the space between the mandible and the zygomatic arch, facilitating needle insertion.

The structures that could potentially be injured with this needle trajectory include the mandibular branch of the trigeminal nerve and the internal maxillary artery and its branches, including the middle meningeal artery. The needle passes through or in between the pterygoid plexus of veins, which is found partly between the temporalis and lateral pterygoid and partly between the two pterygoid muscles. The origin of the maxillary artery from the external carotid artery is embedded in the parotid gland posterior to the neck of the mandible. The mandibular part of the artery runs horizontally forward along the

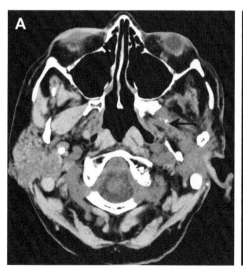
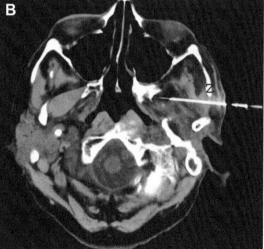

Fig. 1. Subzygomatic approach. (*A*) CT scan shows a partly calcified mass (*black arrow*) in relation to the pterygoid plates. (*B*) CT scan shows a biopsy needle that was inserted inferior to the posterior part of the zygomatic arch (z) and advanced medially into the mass.

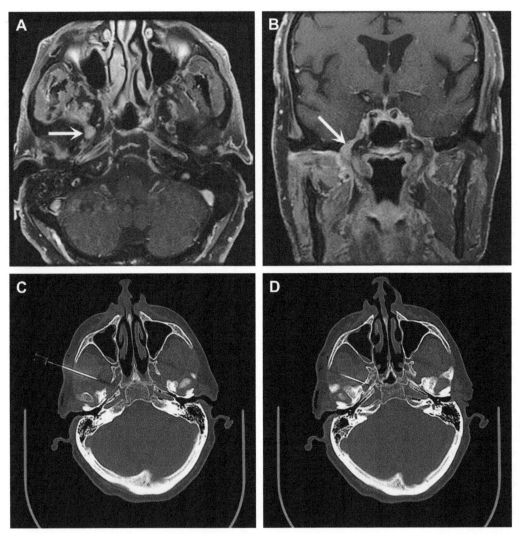

Fig. 2. Subzygomatic approach. Axial (*A*) and coronal (*B*) MR images show a soft tissue mass (*white arrow*) extending inferiorly through a widened foramen ovale along the V3 nerve into the upper portion of the masticator space. (*C*) CT scan shows the biopsy needle inserted at a level caudal to the zygomatic arch. The needle was advanced in a cranial direction using the triangulation method. (*D*) CT scan at a more cranial level shows the needle tip in the lesion.

medial surface of the ramus and the pterygoid part ascends forward and medially, located either superficial (60%) or deep (40%) to the lateral pterygoid muscle, to enter the pterygopalatine fossa through the pterygomaxillary fissure. The mandibular part gives origin to the middle meningeal artery, which ascends in the posterior part of the sigmoid notch deep to the lateral pterygoid muscle to enter the foramen spinosum. After exiting the cranial cavity through the foramen ovale, the mandibular nerve descends in the posterior part of the intercondylar notch (medial to the lateral pterygoid muscle and anterior to the neck of the mandible) to reach the inner surface of the mandibular ramus. However,

the risk of major injury to the vessels or the nerves is extremely low.

Retromandibular (Transparotid) Approach

Lesions in the deep parotid space, parapharyngeal space, pharyngeal mucosal space, and lower part of the retropharyngeal space are accessible via a retromandibular approach. This approach can also be used for targeting lesions in the carotid sheath, if the vessels are displaced medially by the mass.

With this approach, the needle is inserted posterior to the mandible and anterior to the mastoid process and advanced through the parotid gland (Fig. 3). The external carotid artery and the retromandibular vein, which are located within the parotid gland immediately posterior to the mandibular ramus, should be avoided. The external carotid artery, after exiting the carotid sheath, turns laterally and passes anterior to the posterior belly of the digastric muscle to reach the parotid gland. Within the substance of the parotid gland, it is located medial to the retromandibular vein, and ascends behind the condyle before dividing into the superficial temporal and maxillary arteries. The facial nerve as it courses through the parotid gland is located lateral to the retromandibular vein. The needle should be kept anterior to the styloid process to avoid injury to the internal carotid artery, which is located posterior to the styloid process. Occasionally, however, medial displacement of the carotid vessels by mass lesions may allow the needle to be advanced posterior to the styloid process.

The presence of osseous structures such as the styloid and the mastoid processes, and mandible, does not allow much room for needle angulation, making it difficult to access the skull base, the prevertebral space, the cervical spine, and portions of the retropharyngeal space with this approach (Fig. 4).[19] Large-caliber needles should not be used with this approach because of the potential risk of injury to the facial nerve.

Paramaxillary (Retromaxillary, Buccal Space) Approach

The paramaxillary approach offers safe access to lesions in the infrazygomatic portion of the masticator space, the posterior portions of the parapharyngeal and pharyngeal mucosal spaces, the carotid sheath space, and the deep portion of the parotid space.[20,21] It is particularly useful for lesions in the lateral part of the retropharyngeal (eg, lateral retropharyngeal node of Rouviere) space and prevertebral portion of the perivertebral space because these lesions are difficult to access by other approaches. This approach also allows access to anterior C1 and C2 lesions, and foramen ovale and other skull base lesions.[19,22] In patients with trigeminal neuralgia, the paramaxillary approach is used for needle placement through the foramen ovale into the Gasserian ganglion for the purpose of chemical, mechanical, or thermal neurolysis.

For this transfacial approach, the needle is inserted inferior to the zygomatic process of the maxilla and advanced posteriorly through the buccal space between the maxilla (alveolar ridge or sinus) and mandible. The needle passes through the buccinator muscle or anterior portion of the masseter muscle or between them. The needle is advanced through the lateral and medial pterygoid muscles and the parapharyngeal space for accessing lesions in the retropharyngeal and carotid space (Fig. 5), and C1 and C2 lesions

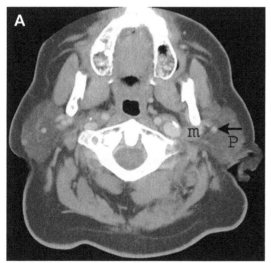
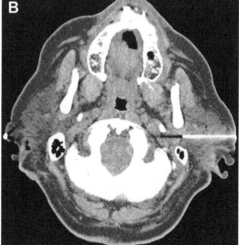

Fig. 3. Retromandibular approach. (A) CT scan shows a mass (m) in the deep parotid space. Note the presence of external carotid artery and retromandibular vein (*arrow*) in the anterior portion of the parotid gland (P). (B) CT scan shows the biopsy needle inserted through the parotid gland and advanced posterior to the vessels into the mass.

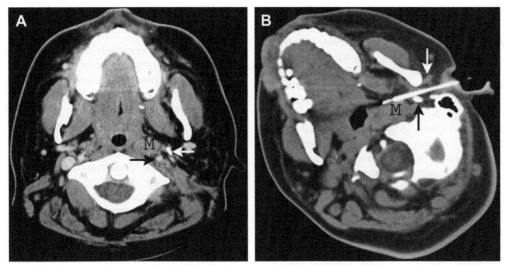

Fig. 4. Retromandibular approach. (*A*) CT scan shows retropharyngeal mass (M). Needle placement posterior the styloid process (*white arrow*) is not possible because of the presence of the internal carotid artery (*black arrow*) directly lateral to the mass. (*B*) Presence of vessels (*white arrow*) in the parotid gland and the styloid process (*black arrow*) limits the needle angulation, restricting access to the mass (M).

(Fig. 6). Foramen ovale and other skull base lesions can be accessed either by using a cranial needle angulation or by causing mild hyperextension of the neck, which brings the skull base lesions and the skin entry site into the same axial plane (see Fig. 5).

The needle trajectory and angulation with the paramaxillary approach is limited by adjacent bones, such as the posterolateral wall of the maxillary antrum, the alveolar ridge, the lateral pterygoid plate, and the anterior margin of the mandibular ramus. In patients with a large maxillary antrum, the space between the maxilla and the mandible may be very narrow, limiting needle placement.

Care should be taken to avoid the facial artery, as it courses in the buccal space The maxillary nerve and its main branches, which course downward in the pterygopalatine fossa, are protected from inadvertent needle injury by the pterygoid plates. It is important to avoid the carotid artery;

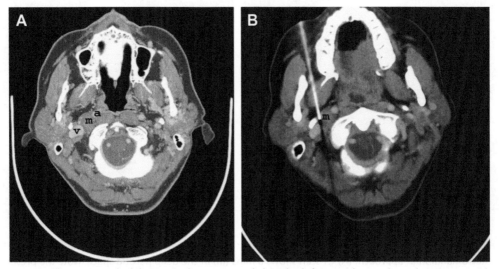

Fig. 5. Paramaxillary approach. (*A*) CT scan shows a mass (m) in the left carotid space lateral to the carotid artery (a) and medial to the jugular vein (v). (*B*) CT scan shows the needle passing through the masticator and parapharyngeal spaces into the mass (m). Contrast was injected to visualize the vessels before obtaining biopsy samples.

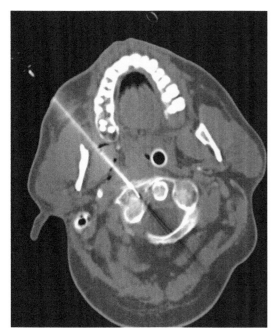

Fig. 6. Paramaxillary approach. CT scan shows the biopsy needle advanced through the masticator and parapharyngeal spaces, and through the prevertebral muscles into a lesion in the lateral mass of atlas.

contrast administration may occasionally be required to visualize the artery, especially when placing a needle in lesions in the carotid sheath space (see **Fig. 5**), the retropharyngeal and prevertebral spaces, and C1 and C2. Other structures that are present in the needle path and could

potentially be injured with this approach include the internal maxillary artery and its branches, the pterygoid venous plexus, branches of the mandibular and maxillary nerves, and the external carotid artery, as it courses laterally deep to the lateral pterygoid muscle. Using a Hawkins-Akins needle (Meditech, Westwood, MA) with a blunt-tip stylet as the outer guiding needle decreases the risk of injury to the vessels and nerves in these spaces.[19,23,24]

Submastoid (Retroparotid) Approach

The submastoid approach can be used for accessing carotid sheath lesions that displace the carotid artery in a medial direction.[19] Lesions in the anterolateral portion of the perivertebral space that displace the carotid sheath anteriorly and the lesions in the parapharyngeal space can also be accessed with this approach. With the patient in a prone position or in a supine position and the head turned to the contralateral side, the needle is inserted inferior to the mastoid tip and advanced anteriorly and medially, and occasionally cranially through the sternocleidomastoid muscle (**Fig. 7**). The needle passes posterior to the parotid gland with this approach and hence there is no risk of damage to the intraparotid vessels, or the facial nerve.

The major structure at risk of injury with this approach is the vertebral artery at the C1–C2 level. After exiting the C2 foramen, the vertebral artery turns outward to reach the external aspect of the lateral mass of C2 and runs cranially along the

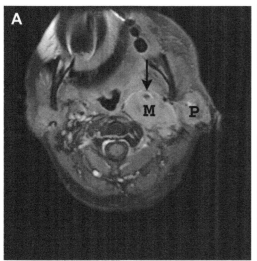

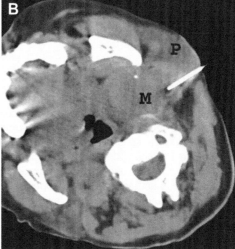

Fig. 7. Submastoid approach. (A) MR shows large mass (M) in the left carotid space encasing the carotid artery (arrow). The parotid gland (P) is immediately lateral to the mass. (B) CT scan with the patient's head turned to the contralateral side shows the biopsy needle passing posterior to the parotid gland into the mass (M). The needle was inserted at a level 1 cm below the tip of the mastoid process (not seen in the image).

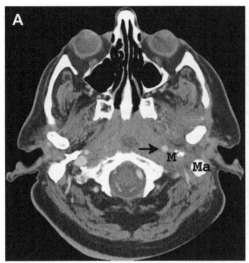
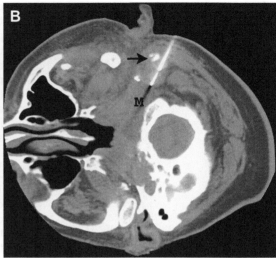

Fig. 8. Retromastoid approach. (*A*) CT scan shows an infiltrating mass (M) in the left carotid space with anterior displacement of the internal carotid artery (*arrow*). The tip of the mastoid (Ma) is present immediately lateral to the mass. (*B*) With the patient in a supine position and the head turned to the contralateral side, the needle was inserted posterior to the mastoid (*arrow*) and advanced in an anterior and medial direction into the mass lesion (M).

lateral mass of C2 before it enters the C1 foramen. The artery then exits the C1 foramen and turns posteriorly to course along the upper surface of the C1 lamina. Administration of contrast medium can be used to visualize the vertebral artery.

Retromastoid Approach

The retromastoid approach can also be occasionally used for biopsy of carotid sheath lesions. With the patient in a prone position or in a supine position and the head turned to the contralateral side, the needle is inserted posterior to the mastoid and advanced in an anterior and medial direction (Fig. 8). Care should be taken to avoid injury to the vertebral and carotid arteries.

Transoral Approach

The transoral approach can be used for percutaneous access to lesions in the retropharyngeal space, the prevertebral part of the perivertebral space, and also for lesions involving the anterior portions of the C1 and C2 vertebrae, including the odontoid.[19,25] The use of this approach requires general anesthesia. A mouth opener is applied and the uvula is pushed away with a retractor or a nasal tube. The posterior pharyngeal wall is sprayed and infiltrated with local anesthetic. The needle is inserted through the posterior pharyngeal mucosa, and is advanced posteriorly through the retropharyngeal space and prevertebral muscles toward the target lesion (Fig. 9). This is a relatively safe approach because no

important structure lies between the posterior pharyngeal wall and the bone. Use of antibiotics is recommended because of difficulty in maintaining a sterile field with the transoral approach.

Posterior Approach

Lesions involving the spinous process, lamina, and articular pillar of the upper cervical vertebrae, the

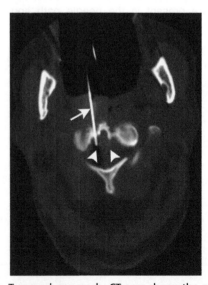

Fig. 9. Transoral approach. CT scan shows the needle (*arrow*) inserted through an open mouth and advanced through the retropharyngeal and prevertebral tissues into a soft tissue mass (*arrowheads*) involving the tip of the odontoid and the anterior arch of atlas.

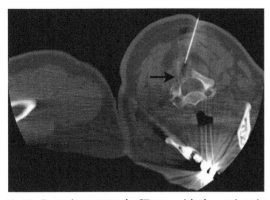

Fig. 10. Posterior approach. CT scan with the patient in the prone position shows the needle that was advanced through the posterior paravertebral muscles for biopsy of a lytic lesion (*arrow*) involving the spinous process and lamina of the C2 vertebra.

occipital condyles, and posterior and lateral portions of the perivertebral space can be accessed by a direct posterior approach (**Fig. 10**). In patients with Arnold's neuralgia, a posterior approach is used for needle placement for anesthetic blockage of the greater occipital nerve. A posterior approach also can be used for sampling lateral masses involving C1 and C2, provided care is taken to identify and avoid the vertebral artery (**Fig. 11**). The vertebral artery, after exiting the C1 foramen, courses posteriorly along the upper surface of the C1 lamina; hence, the needle should be advanced under the lamina, not above it. If

necessary, intravenous administration of contrast medium can be used to help identify the vertebral artery.

APPROACHES USED FOR PERCUTANEOUS ACCESS IN THE INFRAHYOID NECK

The approaches used for percutaneous access in the infrahyoid portion of the neck include the anterolateral (between the airways and the carotid sheath), posterolateral (posterior to the carotid sheath), and direct posterior approaches.[16,26–28]

Anterolateral Approach (Between the Carotid Sheath and Airway)

The anterolateral approach allows access to lesions in the retrotracheal, paraesophageal, and anterior perivertebral spaces. This approach also permits needle placement in bodies of the cervical vertebrae, which can be used for biopsies or for vertebroplasty procedures. Access to the intervertebral disc for biopsy or for discography is possible with this approach, because the disc is not hidden by the uncovertebral joint, which is located more posterolaterally.[16,26–28] Lesions involving the transverse process of the vertebrae can also be reached with this approach as long as the vertebral artery is not in the needle path. This approach has also been used for lower cervical sympathetic chain block.

The needle is inserted adjacent to the medial border of the sternocleidomastoid muscle and advanced posteromedially between the airway and the carotid space (**Figs. 12** and **13**). Manual lateral retraction of the carotid sheath and the sternocleidomastoid muscle can be used to facilitate needle placement. Some authors recommend administration of intravenous atropine to minimize the possibility of a vasovagal response from

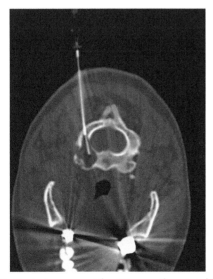

Fig. 11. Posterior approach. CT scan shows a biopsy needle advanced by a posterior approach into a lytic lesion involving the body and lateral mass of C2 vertebra.

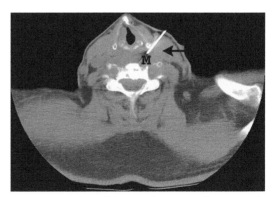

Fig. 12. Anterolateral approach. CT scan shows needle inserted through the medial part of the sternocleidomastoid muscle and advanced between the airway and the carotid sheath (*arrow*) into a prevertebral soft tissue mass (M).

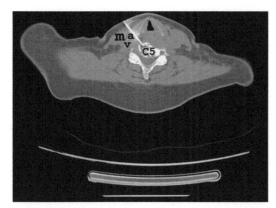

Fig.13. Anterolateral approach. CT scan shows a biopsy needle inserted medial to the sternocleidomastoid muscle (m) and advanced between the thyroid cartilage and the common carotid artery (a) and internal jugular vein (v) for biopsy of a lytic lesion of C5 vertebral body.

compression of the carotid body. Care should be taken to avoid the hypopharynx and especially the pyriform fossa and the esophagus. The esophagus lies to the left of the spine at the level of C7 in most individuals. The needle should not be placed too close to the lateral aspect of the vertebral body because the vertebral artery, in between the foramina in the transverse processes, is located immediately lateral to the mid or posterior part of the vertebral body or disc. Use of intermittent CT scans to check the needle trajectory can prevent the needle from entering the neural foramina, which are directed in an anterolateral direction. Furthermore, the presence of the carotid sheath tends to keep the needle pointed medially and away from the neural foramen and the vertebral artery. Although other structures, including the superior and middle thyroid vessels, the superior and inferior laryngeal nerves, the loop of the hypoglossal nerve, and the cervical ganglia of the sympathetic system, are present in the potential needle path, use of small-caliber needles is unlikely to result in serious injury to these blood vessels or nerves.

Posterolateral Approach (Posterior to the Carotid Sheath)

The posterolateral approach is used for accessing lesions in the prevertebral and lateral paraspinal portions of the perivertebral space, retropharyngeal space, and the posterior cervical space. Lower cervical vertebral lesions that involve the transverse process, pedicle, articular pillar, or lamina can also be accessed by this approach. This approach can also be used for needle placement

in the cervical neural foramina for selective nerve root blocks, and for stellate ganglion or lower cervical sympathetic neurolysis. Because of the presence of large articular masses, uncovertebral joints, and posterior elements in the cervical region, this approach does not allow easy access to the vertebral bodies and the disc spaces.

With the patient in the supine, prone, or lateral decubitus position, the needle is inserted through the sternocleidomastoid muscle and the posterior cervical space and advanced posterior to the carotid sheath (**Fig. 14**). Depending on the axial level in the neck (upper versus lower infrahyoid), the patient's position, and the size and location of the carotid sheath, the needle may be advanced anteromedially or posteromedially. The soft tissues overlying the clavicles and shoulder may interfere with needle placement in the lower neck, particularly in patients with prominent clavicles and short necks. The lowering of the ipsilateral arm and shoulder results in caudal displacement of the clavicle allowing needle placement without osseous interposition. Alternatively, an out-of-plane angled approach with a caudal needle angulation can be used in this situation: the needle is inserted in a plane cranial to the level of the target lesion and advanced caudally and medially (**Fig. 15**).

With this approach, the vertebral artery is the structure most vulnerable to injury during the biopsy, especially at levels between the transverse foramina, where the vessel is located lateral to the vertebral body and disc. Also, a needle inserted behind the carotid sheath and advanced

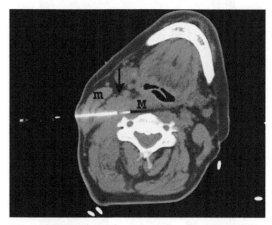

Fig. 14. Posterolateral approach. CT scan shows a biopsy needle inserted through the posterior part of the sternocleidomastoid muscle (m) and advanced in a medial direction. The needle passes posterior to the carotid sheath vessels (*arrow*) into a prevertebral mass (M).

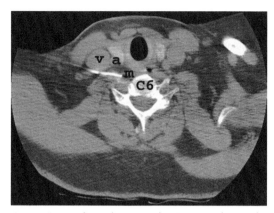

Fig. 15. Posterolateral approach. CT scan shows the biopsy needle in a prevertebral mass (m) at the C6 level. The needle was inserted at a more cranial level, directed caudally and advanced posterior to the internal jugular vein (v) and the common carotid artery (a). The needle stays anterior to the expected location of the vertebral artery.

posteromedially toward a lesion involving the seventh cervical vertebra can potentially injure the vertebral artery. It is important to review MR or contrast-enhanced CT images before placing the needle to avoid puncturing an aberrant or tortuous vertebral artery. Furthermore, a small-caliber needle puncture of the brachial or cervical plexus as it runs between the scalene muscles is not dangerous, although it may cause transient pain.[28]

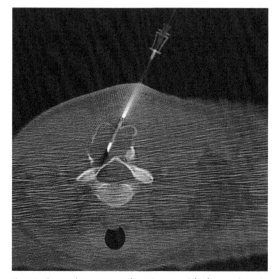

Fig. 16. Posterior approach. CT scan with the patient in the prone position shows the needle passing through the posterior paravertebral muscles into a lytic process involving the spinous process of a cervical vertebra.

Posterior Approach

The posterior approach is used for accessing lesions involving the spinous process, lamina, and articular pillars and processes of the lower cervical vertebrae plus lesions in the posterior and lateral paraspinal portions of the perivertebral space (Fig. 16). Sublaminar epidural steroid injections and facet joint injections in the cervical region are also performed with a posterior approach. With the patient in the prone or lateral decubitus position, the needle is advanced through the posterior paraspinal muscles toward the target lesion. Risk of injury to major vessels or nerves with this approach is extremely low.

SUMMARY

We review the various approaches used for image-guided percutaneous needle placement for diagnostic and therapeutic procedures in the head and neck region and discuss the anatomic and technical aspects and the advantages and limitations of each approach.

REFERENCES

1. Abemayor E, Ljung BM, Ward PH, et al. CT-directed fine needle aspiration biopsies of masses in the head and neck. Laryngoscope 1985;95:1382–6.
2. Abrahams JJ. Mandibular sigmoid notch: a window for CT-guided biopsies of lesions in the peripharyngeal and skull base regions. Radiology 1998;208: 695–9.
3. DelGaudio JM, Dillard DG, Albritton FD, et al. Computed tomography–guided needle biopsy of head and neck lesions. Arch Otolaryngol Head Neck Surg 2000;126:366–70.
4. Fried MP, Hsu L, Jolesz FA. Interactive magnetic resonance imaging-guided biopsy in the head and neck: initial patient experience. Laryngoscope 1998;108:488–93.
5. Gatenby RA, Mulhern CB Jr, Strawitz J. CT-guided percutaneous biopsies of head and neck masses. Radiology 1983;146:717–9.
6. Merkle EM, Lewin JS, Aschoff AJ, et al. Percutaneous magnetic resonance image-guided biopsy and aspiration in the head and neck. Laryngoscope 2000;110:382–5.
7. Sack MJ, Weber RS, Weinstein GS, et al. Image-guided fine-needle aspiration of the head and neck: five years' experience. Arch Otolaryngol Head Neck Surg 1998;124:1155–61.
8. Sherman PM, Yousem DM, Loevner LA. CT-guided aspirations in the head and neck: assessment of the first 216 cases. AJNR Am J Neuroradiol 2004; 25:1603–7.

9. Harnsberger HR, Osborn AG. Differential diagnosis of head and neck lesions based on their space of origin. 1. The suprahyoid part of the neck. AJR Am J Roentgenol 1991;157:147–54.

10. Smoker WR, Harnsberger HR. Differential diagnosis of head and neck lesions based on their space of origin. 2. The infrahyoid portion of the neck. AJR Am J Roentgenol 1991;157:155–9.

11. Ridder GJ, Technau-Ihling K, Boedeker CC. Ultrasound-guided cutting needle biopsy in the diagnosis of head and neck masses. Laryngoscope 2005;115:376–7.

12. Screaton NJ, Berman LH, Grant JW. Head and neck lymphadenopathy: evaluation with US-guided cutting-needle biopsy. Radiology 2002;224:75–81.

13. Screaton NJ, Berman LH, Grant JW. US-guided core-needle biopsy of the thyroid gland. Radiology 2003;226:827–32.

14. Kornblum MB, Wesolowski DP, Fischgrund JS, et al. Computed tomography-guided biopsy of the spine. A review of 103 patients. Spine 1998;23:81–5.

15. Ljung BM, Larsson SG, Hanafee W. Computed tomography-guided aspiration cytologic examination in head and neck lesions. Arch Otolaryngol 1984;110:604–7.

16. Tampieri D, Weill A, Melanson D, et al. Percutaneous aspiration biopsy in cervical spine lytic lesions. Indications and technique. Neuroradiology 1991;33:43–7.

17. Lewin JS, Nour SG, Duerk JL. Magnetic resonance image-guided biopsy and aspiration. Top Magn Reson Imaging 2000;11:173–83.

18. Walker AT, Chaloupka JC, Putman CM, et al. Sentinel transoral hemorrhage from a pseudoaneurysm of the internal maxillary artery: a complication of CT-guided biopsy of the masticator space. AJNR Am J Neuroradiol 1996;17:377–81.

19. Gupta S, Henningsen JA, Wallace MJ, et al. Percutaneous biopsy of head and neck lesions with CT guidance: various approaches and relevant anatomic and technical considerations. Radiographics 2007;27:371–90.

20. Esposito MB, Arrington JA, Murtagh FR, et al. Anterior approach for CT-guided biopsy of skull base and parapharyngeal space lesions. J Comput Assist Tomogr 1996;20:739–41.

21. Tu AS, Geyer CA, Mancall AC, et al. The buccal space: a doorway for percutaneous CT-guided biopsy of the parapharyngeal region. AJNR Am J Neuroradiol 1998;19:728–31.

22. Dresel SH, Mackey JK, Lufkin RB, et al. Meckel cave lesions: percutaneous fine-needle-aspiration biopsy cytology. Radiology 1991;179:579–82.

23. Akins EW, Hawkins IF Jr, Mladinich C, et al. The blunt needle: a new percutaneous access device. AJR Am J Roentgenol 1989;152:181–2.

24. Mukherji SK, Turetsky D, Tart RP, et al. A technique for core biopsies of head and neck masses. AJNR Am J Neuroradiol 1994;15:518–20.

25. Patil AA. Transoral stereotactic biopsy of the second cervical vertebral body: case report with technical note. Neurosurgery 1989;25:999–1001 [discussion: 1001–2].

26. Kang M, Gupta S, Khandelwal N, et al. CT-guided fine-needle aspiration biopsy of spinal lesions. Acta Radiol 1999;40:474–8.

27. Kattapuram SV, Rosenthal DI. Percutaneous biopsy of the cervical spine using CT guidance. AJR Am J Roentgenol 1987;149:539–41.

28. Ottolenghi CE, Schajowicz F, Deschant FA. Aspiration biopsy of the cervical spine. Technique and results in thirty-four cases. J Bone Joint Surg Am 1964;46:715–33.

Percutaneous Thermal Ablation in the Head and Neck: Current Role and Future Applications

Gerald Wyse, MB, BCh[a],*, H. Hong, MD[b], Kieran Murphy, MB, BCh[c]

KEYWORDS

- Head and neck cancer
- Percutaneous thermal ablation therapies
- Radiofrequency ablation • Cryoablation

Image-guided ablation therapies are an emerging minimally invasive treatment modality for the treatment of head and neck tumors. These techniques are predominantly used as a palliative treatment of pain and local tumor control in the setting of recurrent head and neck cancers.[1,2] In patients with a head or neck tumor, wide surgical resection offers the best cure. Unfortunately, the majority of patients presents with locally advanced disease and are not good surgical candidates because of their disease extent or poor functional status.[3] In these patients, minimally invasive ablation treatments potentially offer improved quality of life, decreased tumor burden and may increase survival.

Tumor ablation results in the focal destruction of solid tumor by eradicating all viable tumor cells in the area. The head and neck is a unique location with its own inherent risks related to the close proximity of the surrounding anatomical structures. Percutaneous ablation therapies offer potential advantages with minimal damage to surrounding tissue with preservation of surrounding tissue function.

Ablation techniques are most often used in the setting of recurrent disease with a history of previous surgery and or radiation therapy. In this setting, treatments such as repeat surgery, external beam radiation and systemic chemotherapy have poor results in terms of survival and quality of life.[4,5] Scar tissue and loss of the normal anatomical planes makes recurrent surgery challenging with high rates of complications. These common treatments are often toxic with significant effect on swallowing function, speech, cosmetic appearance and poor wound healing.

Ablation techniques such as radiofrequency ablation (RFA) and cryotherapy are in widespread use and have been shown to be successful in the setting of various tumors involving the bone, lung, prostate, kidney, and liver. As compared with repetitive invasive surgery, ablation techniques offer a significant reduction in morbidity and mortality at a much lower procedural cost. Ablations are often carried out as outpatient procedures or with a short hospital stay. There is a minimal incision and no significant blood loss.

Ablative techniques offer an additional treatment option for patients with head and neck cancer. It is critical that these techniques, whether used alone or in combination with other therapies, are used as a consensus derived, multidisciplinary approach to cancer.

TUMORS OF THE HEAD AND NECK: ABLATION TECHNIQUES

As in many medical disciplines, patient selection is critical. Use of ablative techniques in the head and

[a] Division of Interventional Neuroradiology, Department of Radiology, Johns Hopkins University, 600 North Wolfe Street, Baltimore, MD 21287, USA
[b] Division of Interventional Radiology, Department of Radiology, Johns Hopkins Medical Institutions, 600 North Wolfe Street, Baltimore MD 21211, USA
[c] University of Toronto Medical Imaging, 150 College Street, Toronto, Ontario M53 3E2, Canada, USA
* Corresponding author.
E-mail address: gwysel@jhmi.edu (G. Wyse).

neck have been reported in the literature in the setting of squamous cell carcinoma,[1,2] tumors of the oral cavity,[6] paranasal sinuses,[6] thyroid tumors,[7] adenoid cystic carcinoma of the salivary glands,[8] solitary fibrous tumors,[9] and recurrent melanoma.[2] Primary surgical resection, modified neck dissections and external beam radiation remain the pillars of primary treatment for these conditions. Ablative techniques have been shown to be effective as primary treatment in certain subgroups of patients—such as those who are excluded from surgical cure because of significant heart, lung, or liver disease. However, the role of ablative techniques in the setting of primary treatment is currently unproven and all patients should be offered gold standard, first line therapy prior to an ablation procedure.

DIAGNOSTIC WORK-UP AND IMAGING

Clinical evaluation and review of all relevant imaging is imperative prior to any ablation procedure. Patient expectations and clear treatment goals need to be defined. Critical appraisal of all cross-sectional imaging with particular attention to tumor extent and proximity of delicate surrounding structures is essential. Renal function, platelet counts, and coagulation factors are all reviewed. In cases of recurrent thyroid carcinoma, endoscopic examination of the vocal cords is warranted.

Depending on the tumor location, an ablation probe can be inserted percutaneously, transorally, or by an endoscopic guided route. Ablation procedures are commonly performed under CT or ultrasound guidance. The choice of the guiding modality depends on tumor location and operator preference. The key to all ablation techniques is the precise positioning of the ablation probe within the tumor. Multiple probes or overlapping ablation segments ensure eradication of all local tumor cells. Ultrasound is commonly used in the setting of thyroid tumors (Fig. 1A–D). In addition to allowing excellent real-time visualization, ultrasound is better at visualizing ablative zones than CT in the setting of RFA.

CT also provides precise anatomic visualization of the tumor. The use of contrast can aid in tumor visualization and in determining the relationship of the tumor to the adjacent vascular structures. CT fluoroscopy can be used to aid in accurate probe insertion and avoid inadvertent puncture of any vessel or the aerodigestive tract (Fig. 2). Contrast-enhanced CT after the ablation may lead to identification of residual enhancing tumor that can be further ablated in the same treatment setting. There is a role for interventional MR imaging guidance in this field as the thermal imaging capability can define heat distribution and thus allow reduction of inadvertent nerve or other organ injury.

RADIOFREQUENCY ABLATION

The aim is to ablate all viable tumor cells with a small surrounding margin of normal tissue, similar to the concept of clear surgical resection margins. Sterile grounding pads are evenly placed in a position that is easy and convenient to check, they are optimally placed equidistant from the target ablation site to allow equal grounding of thermal energy, usually on both thighs. This helps avoid skin burns. Delicate surrounding visceral or vascular structures can be pushed away from the ablated zone by means of a hydrodissection technique in which a small needle is carefully placed between target tissue and the surrounding vital structures. Intervening space can be increased by the introduction of an insulator such as sterile water, dextrose, air, or carbon dioxide. Saline is a conductor and may increase the size of the ablation zone. An RFA probe consists of an insulated shaft and an active tip. Probes come in varies sizes with multiple tip lengths and configurations. Deployable distal tips with multiple tines are used for large bulky tumors (Fig. 3). These complex shapes allow for large reproducible regions of ablation. Point tips are often used for smaller lesions. Through the probe, there is transmission of low-voltage alternating current that creates ionic agitation, heating, intratumoral hyperthermia, and tumor necrosis. This is referred to as focal coagulative necrosis.[10] Both current and heat decrease exponentially as the distance increases from the active tip of the probe. Ablation temperatures reach 50°C to 100°C. There is a cytotoxic threshold temperature for the tumor cells. Most malignant cells are rapidly destroyed above 50°C. The aim is for the entire tumor to be subject to a cytotoxic temperature. If the tissue surrounding the tip of the probe is overheated, it will vaporize and char. This will decrease the energy absorbed and reduce the size of the surrounding ablation.[11] When tissue reaches in excess of 100°C, it will vaporize with resultant reduced ablation of the surrounding tissue. The impedance or temperature at the probe tip is monitored and the output of the generator is adjusted to prevent vaporization and charring. To avoid charring, probes can have a cooled tip with chilled saline circulating in the shaft of the probe.

In addition, it is important to consider the surrounding tissue and their effect on the ablation zone. Fat insulates an ablation zone, whereas vascular structures decrease the size of the

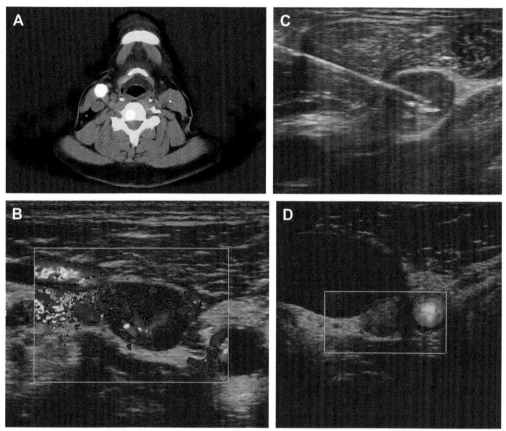

Fig. 1. A 43-year-old man had a history of papillary thyroid carcinoma treated with total thyroidectomy and right modified radial neck dissection. Increasing thyroglobulin levels were noted before this study and there was clinical evidence of recurrent mass. (*A*) Positron emission tomography CT reveals a hypermetabolic node at level II on the right side. (*B*) Ultrasound reveals an enlarged hypervascular node, confirmed on biopsy as recurrent papillary thyroid carcinoma. (*C*) Ultrasound-guided RFA. Two ablations, 1 minute each were performed with temperatures in the high-60°C range. (*D*) Follow-up ultrasound 7 months later shows an echogenic hypovascular shrunken node. Thyroglobulin levels also returned to normal. (*Courtesy of* Damian Dupuy, MD, Providence, RI.)

ablation zone. This heat sink effect occurs when high tissue perfusion from an adjacent vessel results in cooling of the tissue. The flowing blood carries energy away from the ablation zone and reduces the amount of ablated tissue. This can lead to viable tumor surviving an ablation. Portal vein occlusion in an animal model has been used in the liver to reduce the heat sink effect and increase the size of an ablation.[12] Such techniques in the neck and head are likely to lead to higher complication rates and are not advisable. Pharmacological manipulation of blood flow to reduce heat sink may have a future role in ablation techniques.

Slow withdrawal of the RFA needle at an angle of 50° to 70° will help to cauterize the tract. This helps prevent bleeding and may reduce the chances of seeding the tumor along the tract.

In comparison with other modalities, there is reduced blood loss and fewer bleeding complications. On the downside, RFA is associated with significant procedural and post procedural pain.

CRYOABLATION

Similar to RFA, an ablation probe is inserted into a tumor, usually under image guidance. Cryoablation results in formation of a well-defined iceball at the probe tip. With the probe tip embedded in the tumor, the surrounding tissue is destroyed. This iceball delineates the ablation zone. The iceball is easily visualized on both ultrasound and CT. The tip of the ablation probe is cooled by circulation of liquid argon or helium or both. Cryoablation works by extreme tissue cooling resulting in damage to enzymatic systems, proteins, and

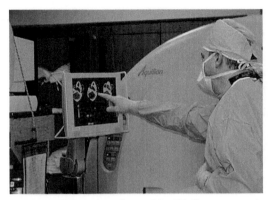

Fig. 2. Real-time imaging with CT fluoroscopy in a patient undergoing RFA of a sarcoma of the zygoma. The patient had a history of radiation therapy for metastatic breast carcinoma. The RFA successfully debulked the tumor improving both pain symptoms and the cosmetic appearance.

membranes. There is intracellular ice formation and extracellular freezing. This causes water to be drawn out of the cell and resultant osmotic dehydration. Cryoablation also results in vascular injury within the tissue. By using a series of freezing and thawing cycles, the tumor cells are destroyed.[13,14]

A variety of factors determines the extent of the tumor kill using this technique. These include: the speed of freezing, the lowest temperature, duration of the lowest temperature, and the tissue inhomogeneity. The size of the iceball is controlled by the rate at which the gas is delivered. Multiple overlapping probes can be used in one ablation to treat large irregular tumors. It is possible to shape the iceball by strategic placement of multiple probes.

The procedure is considerably less painful than RFA because of the anesthetic effect of freezing. Recent reduction in probe size means that there is less concern about hemorrhage. In the head and neck, percutaneous cryoablation has been used in the setting of a fibrous tumor of the buccal space.[9] Cryoablation is in widespread use for the treatment of malignant renal,[15] hepatic,[16] bone[17] tumors, and the prostate.

Cortical bone has poor conductivity and makes RFA less effective when the tumor involves or is adjacent to bone.[18] As a result, tumor at the skull base or involving the vertebral bodies of the cervical spine may at least be theoretically better treated by cryoablation.

THE ABLATION PROCEDURE

Preprocedure planning is essential in the head and neck. Patient eye protection and attention to

pressure points need to be considered. Similar to any head and neck biopsy, manipulation of the patient's head position or angulation of the CT gantry may provide an easy access route. See the article by Gupta elsewhere in this issue for a detailed review of percutaneous approaches to head and neck spaces.

Although practices vary, a large number of head and neck ablations are performed under general anesthesia. This allows precise and accurate ablation probe insertion while protecting the airway. Ablation procedures can be extremely painful with multiple probe insertions, manipulations, and ablation cycles. Smaller lesions can be ablated under conscious sedation with a combination of fentanyl and midazolam. Pulse oximetry, blood pressure, and electrocardiography are monitored throughout the ablation procedure.

All equipment is dry table tested before probe insertion. Connections to RFA generators, generator output or cryoablation gas supply, and output are all confirmed. Intravenous prophylactic antibiotics are administered. Antibiotic use is more theoretical than evidence based, although their use is widespread. The ablation probe or probes are inserted directly into the tumor.

For single probe ablations, the tip is positioned centrally within the tumor. Alternatively, the probe is positioned at one end of the tumor, an ablation cycle is performed, and the probe is repositioned. The cycle is then repeated with multiple overlapping ablative segments. In the setting of cryoablation, multiple overlapping probes are positioned to completely cover and eradicate all tumor cells. Post ablation, the probes are removed and a sterile adhesive dressing applied.

The patient is usually observed for 4 to 6 hours in recovery then discharged home with appropriate analgesia. Overnight observation is recommended for any tumor adjacent to or involving the airway.

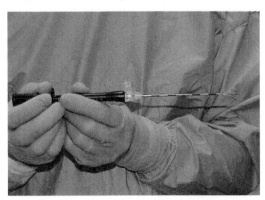

Fig. 3. An RFA probe with a deployable distal tip with multiple tines that is used for large bulky tumors.

Prolonged intubation can be contemplated for any ablation that is close to the airway and there is concern for postablation swelling. Consultation in an anesthesia clinic prior to the planned procedure can mitigate such potential concerns, particularly in the setting of general anesthesia and a high-risk patient. In addition, large tumors may be associated with significant pain post procedure and are best observed overnight. Neck discomfort and soft tissue swelling are common and usually self-limiting after ablation procedures.

ALTERNATIVE AND FUTURE ABLATION TECHNIQUES
Microwave Ablation

Microwave ablation utilizes electromagnetic energy to produce heating and cell death in malignant tissue. Microwave probes allow a large zone of heating without the charring or vaporization problems seen in RFA. Microwave ablation uses percutaneously placed probes within a tumor to focus externally applied energy. There is a theoretical advantage in higher tumor temperatures, reduced heat sink effects, and large zones of achievable ablation.[19,20] Although the current size of the probes at 14 gauge makes them impractical for all but the largest of the head and neck tumors, there are various types of microwave probes available. Similar to some RFA probes, they may consist of an active tip and a saline cooled shaft to prevent thermal injury. Although their use in the head and neck is currently limited, a future reduction in probe size may offer an alternative ablative option for patients with head and neck tumors.

Laser

Laser ablation is possible through a percutaneous approach to a tumor. A coaxial needle is placed within the tumor and a thin flexible optic fiber advanced into the tumor cells. An Nd:YAG laser may be used. The heating of the malignant cells induces coagulation necrosis. Although not currently in use in the head and neck, laser ablation may provide a future treatment option.

MR Imaging-Guided Ultrasound

MR imaging-guided, focused, high-intensity ultrasound has been used successfully as an ablative therapy for uterine fibroids[21] and for bone metastases.[22] Although no current reports of use exist in the head or neck, this technique has exciting clinical applications. A beam of high intensity ultrasound energy is focused on a point. The energy is transmitted transcutaneously without the need for insertion of a probe into the skin. The ultrasound energy is converted into heat and leads to coagulative necrosis. MR imaging is used to define and target the tumor. There is direct feedback of the effectiveness of the ablation therapy. This is performed with MR imaging thermometry. This technique measures real time temperature and has the ability to detect if a cytotoxic temperature has been reached in a tumor. This gives an on-table ability to increase the chance of a successful ablation. As a therapeutic option for patients with cancer, MR imaging thermometry offers one of the most exciting and promising technologies currently being developed for cancer treatment.

Percutaneous Ethanol Injection

This ablation method has been used for small lesions predominately in the setting of locally recurrent papillary thyroid carcinoma. This procedure is often performed under ultrasound with real time visualization of the needle tip within the lesion being critical. Ethanol induces tissue necrosis through cellular dehydration, protein denaturation, and small vessel thrombosis. Percutaneous ethanol injection as a technique is simple, low cost, and easily repeated.[23]

High Intensity Interstitial Ultrasound

High-intensity interstitial ultrasound (HIIU) utilizes multiple individually focused ultrasound elements that are mounted on a single needle. These elements can be controlled to allow conformation of the energy generated to the complex shape of the tumor (**Fig. 4**). At the author's institution, we have studied this technique in an in vivo rabbit model in which we had grown VX2 tumors in the vertebra and paravertebral musculature (K. Murphy, unpublished data, 2007) (**Fig. 5**A). Within 6 weeks, we were able to grow a tumor capable of causing cord compression. We confirmed the ability to control the energy distribution by placing multiple thermocouples around the therapeutic needle (**Fig. 5**B). We then confirmed the ability of the technique to kill the margins of the tumor with pathologic examination. Our objective is to develop a device that can be used kill tumor margins close to critical structures while preserving the margins.

FOLLOW-UP OR RETREATMENT

Both short- and long-term imaging follow-up are essential. This ensures the stability of a lesion and will detect residual or recurrent disease at an early stage. Contrast-enhanced CT or MR imaging is typically used, but positron emission

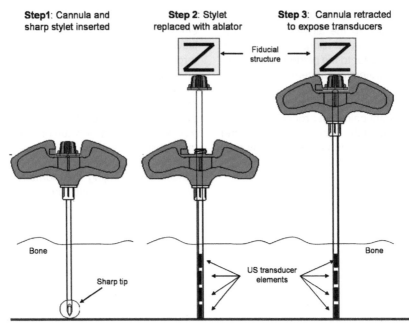

Step 1: Cannula and sharp stylet inserted

Step 2: Stylet replaced with ablator

Step 3: Cannula retracted to expose transducers

Fiducial structure

Bone

Bone

Sharp tip

US transducer elements

Fig. 4. HIIU ablation devices are composed of multiple high-energy ultrasound elements that can be individually focused and set at different ablation energies. The larger the guiding needle, the greater the number and diameter of ablation elements that can be used. This illustration shows a four-element HIIU device passed through an 11-gauge vertebroplasty needle.

tomography/CT (PET/CT) may be helpful in the setting of previous surgery or radiation therapy. Follow-up cross-sectional imaging typically shows a central nonenhancing core representing the ablated area. A rim of smooth, thin enhancing tissue is commonly seen around the site of ablation for several weeks to months, consistent with granulation tissue. Biopsy is advisable for thickened or nodular enhancing tissue. Follow-up imaging on ultrasound will show decreased vascularity with ablated lesions becoming hyperechoic. Reduction in tumor volume will take several months.

COMPLICATIONS

Ablation techniques intentionally destroy a sphere or cylinder of tissue surrounding the ablation probe. Ablation zones do not respect tissue planes and can damage surrounding structures such as the nerves, blood vessels, and the aerodigestive tract. Ablation zones in the head and neck can be quite different from those in the rest of the body, especially the liver. Overall, the liver is a large forgiving organ in relation to ablation techniques. Care is needed in the head and neck to avoid faster and larger ablations zones with resultant complications.

Heating can result in skin burns and cellulites. This is usually self-limited, although skin breakdown can occur. Vascular structures are somewhat protected by fast-flowing blood. However, carotid blowout[6] and delay stroke[1] have been described. Fistula formation is a real concern and has devastating consequences on quality of life. Hoarseness post ablation is often a sign of recurrent laryngeal nerve injury and is an important consideration in thyroid and parathyroid ablations.[7] Extreme care is needed to ensure the ablative probe is as far as possible from all these delicate surrounding structures—especially when prior surgery or radiation has altered the anatomy.

Fever after the procedure is common. A postablation syndrome can occur which is often mild in comparison with a tumor lyses syndrome. These post ablation syndromes usually resolve with supportive measures, although a severe form called cryoshock consisting of coagulopathy, renal, and pulmonary injury has been described.[24] In the case of a nonresolving fever, abscess formation is a consideration. Antibiotic coverage, cultures and reimaging should be considered when the fever persists.

FUTURE RESEARCH DIRECTIONS

There is currently no evidence to support ablation techniques over primary surgical resection and radiotherapy. Although anecdotal evidence suggests a larger role for ablative therapies, there is a need for, first, further prospective studies to

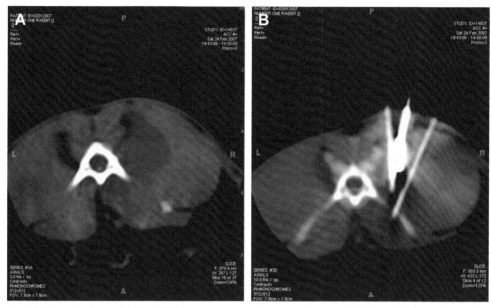

Fig. 5. A rabbit was implanted with a VX2 tumor as a cord compression model. This rabbit was then successfully treated with HIIU. Pathologic examination confirmed the ability of this technique to kill the margins of the tumor. (A) Unenhanced CT image reveals a right-sided paraspinal tumor in the rabbit. (B) CT-fluoroscopy image shows a central large HIIU needle and its elements. On either side are the thermocouples placed to measure heat distribution and to monitor the physician's ability to aim the ablative energy one way or the other. This control will help to ensure complete tumor kill with minimal damage to surrounding structures. A, anterior; L, left; P, posterior; R, right.

determine their efficacy and safety and, ultimately, large randomized prospective trials to compare the efficacy of ablation and surgical techniques.

There is the possibility of improved patient outcomes with combined therapies including radiation and chemotherapy. These treatments may make tissue more responsive to ablation techniques. Similar to approaches used in liver tumors, a combined strategy involving intra-arterial chemoembolization and ablation techniques may improve outcomes for head and neck cancers. Direct injection of liposomal chemotherapeutic agents during ablation procedures have been shown to a have potential synergy in liver tumor and may be a possibility.[25]

REFERENCES

1. Owen RP, Silver CE, Radvikumar TS, et al. Techniques for radiofrequency ablation of head and neck tumors. Arch Otolaryngol Head Neck Surg 2004;130(1):52–6.

2. Liukko T, Makitie AA, Markkola A, et al. Radiofrequency induced thermotherapy: an alternative palliative treatment modality in head and neck cancer. Eur Arch Otorhinolaryngol 2006;263(6):532–6.

3. Vokes EE, Weichselbaum RR, Lippman SM, et al. Head and neck cancer. N Engl J Med 1993;328:184–94.

4. Tupchong L, Scott CB, Blitzer PH, et al. Randomized study of preoperative versus postoperative radiation therapy in advanced head and neck carcinoma; long-term follow-up of RTOG study 73-03. Int J Radiat Oncol Biol Phys 1991;20(1):21–8.

5. Silver CE, Owen RP. Morbidity of salvage surgery for recurrent head and neck cancer. In: Proceedings on head and neck cancer. Pittsburgh (PA): American Head and Neck Society; 2000. p. 569–75.

6. Brook AL, Gold MM, Miller TS, et al. CT-guided radiofrequency ablation in the palliative treatment of recurrent advanced head and neck malignancies. J Vasc Interv Radiol 2008;19(5):725–35.

7. Dupuy DE, Monchik JM, Decrea C, et al. Radiofrequency ablation of regional recurrence from well-differentiated thyroid malignancy. Surgery 2001;130(6):971–7.

8. Bui Q, Dupuy DE. Percutaneous CT-guided radiofrequency ablation of an adenoid cystic carcinoma of the head and neck. AJR Am J Roentgenol 2002;179:1333–5.

9. Schirmang TC, Davis LM, Nigiri PT, et al. Solitary fibrous tumor of the buccal space; treatment with percutaneous cryoablation. AJNR Am J Neuroradiol 2007;28(9):1728–30.

10. Cosman E, Nashold B, Ovelman-Levitt J. Theoretical aspects of radiofrequency lesions in the dorsal root entry zone. Neurosurgery 1984;15:945–50.

11. Goldberg SN, Gazelle GC, Halpern EF, et al. Radio-frequency tissue ablation; importance of local temperature along the electrode tip exposure in determining lesion shape and size. Acad Radiol 1996;3:212–8.

12. Patterson EJ, Scudamore CH, Owen DA, et al. Radiofrequency ablation of porcine liver in vivo: effects of blood flow and treatment time on lesion size. Ann Surg 1998;227:559–65.

13. Cooper IS. Cryogenic surgery: a new method of destruction or extiration of benign of malignant tissue. N Engl J Med 1963;268:743–9.

14. Rubinsky B, Lee CY, Bastacty J, et al. The process of freezing and the mechanism of damage during hepatic cryosurgery. Cryobiology 1990;27:85–97.

15. Shingleton WB, Sewell PE Jr. Percutaneous renal tumor cryoablation with magnetic resonance imaging guidance. J Urol 2001;165:773–6.

16. KerKar S, Carlin AM, Sohn RL, et al. Long-term follow up and prognostic factor for cryotherapy of malignant liver tumors. Surgery 2004;136:770–9.

17. Callstrom MR, Atwell TD, Charboneau JW, et al. Painful image-guided cryoablation—prospective trial interim analysis. Radiology 2006;241:572–80.

18. Dupuy DE, Hong R, Oliver B, et al. Radiofrequency ablation of spinal tumors: temperature distribution in the spinal canal. AJR Am J Roentgenol 2000; 175:1263–6.

19. Haemmerich D, Laeseke PF. Thermal tumour ablation: devices, clinical applications and future directions. Int J Hyperthermia 2005;21:755–60.

20. Skinner MG, Lizuka MN, Kolios MC, et al. A theoretical comparison of energy sources—microwave, ultrasound and laser—for interstitial thermal therapy. Phys Med Biol 1998;43:3535–47.

21. Tempany CM, Stewart EA, McDannold N, et al. MR imaging-guided focused ultrasound surgery of uterine leiomyomas: a feasibility study. Radiology 2003;226:897–905.

22. Gianfelice D, Gupta C, Kucharczyk W, et al. Palliative treatment of painful bone metastases with MR imaging-guided focused ultrasound. Radiology 2008;249:355–63.

23. Lewis BD, Hay ID, Charboneau JW, et al. Percutaneous ethanol injection for treatment of cervical lymph node metastases in patients with papillary thyroid carcinoma. AJR Am J Roentgenol 2002; 178(3):699–704.

24. Georgiades C, Hong K, Geschwind JF, et al. Short & long term complications from percutaneous renal cryoablation. Risks & mitigating actions. J Vasc Interv Radiol 2008;19(2):40–1.

25. Goldberg SN, Kamel IR, Kruskal JB, et al. Radiofrequency ablation of hepatic tumors: increased tumor destruction with adjuvant liposomal doxorubicin therapy. AJR Am J Roentgenol 2002;179(1):93–101.

Developmental Anatomy, Angiography, and Clinical Implications of Orbital Arterial Variations Involving the Stapedial Artery

Philippe Gailloud, MD*, Lydia Gregg, MA, Diego San Millán Ruiz, MD

KEYWORDS

- Ophthalmic artery • Orbital arteries • Anatomy
- Embolization • Dangerous anastomoses

Over the past 200 years, classical anatomists have provided a detailed description of the arterial collateral pathways that can be found in the head and neck. The small branches building this intricate arterial network often are difficult to access, as they are located near or within the skull base. They have been revealed, one at a time, at the price of precise but painstaking anatomic dissections. The arterial map inherited from the anatomists recently has been put to the test with detailed high-resolution vascular imaging. Superselective angiography, in particular, has helped rediscover the complexity of the craniocervical arterial network under normal and pathologic conditions.[1,2] The concept of dangerous collaterals or dangerous anastomoses was born with the advent of endovascular therapy. Until then, the arterial network of the skull base had been seen as a safety mechanism bringing relief to areas that had lost their primary source of blood supply (eg, the classic cerebral collateral supply through the ophthalmic artery [OA] in case of proximal carotid occlusion). With the introduction of transarterial embolization, these beneficial pathways also have become a potential source of procedural complications, mostly by inadvertent passage of embolic material into branches supplying important structures, such as the eye or the brain. In addition to confirming the accuracy of anatomic knowledge, superselective angiography has shown that most of the so-called dangerous collaterals, although consistently present under normal and abnormal conditions, may become angiographically conspicuous only under particular hemodynamic circumstances. For example, a connection between the occipital artery and the vertebral artery may "appear" (ie, become detectable) during the course of an embolization dealing with a distal occipital artery lesion. Such a phenomenon emphasizes the need for strict embolization techniques and the necessity to master the complex anatomy of these dangerous connections. Although dangerous anastomoses of the skull base are well described in the literature,[2,3] the variations and collateral pathways related to the orbital arteries often have been overlooked or misunderstood, in spite of their importance for safe extraorbital embolization procedures. This article presents a review of the normal orbital arterial vascularization and its principal variations, with particular emphasis placed on abnormal pathways involving residual segments of the stapedial artery.

ARTERIAL VASCULARIZATION OF THE ORBIT
Development

The arterial supply to the orbit combines, in its normal adult configuration, vascular elements

Division of Interventional Neuroradiology, Department of Radiology, The Johns Hopkins Hospital, 600 N. Wolfe Street, Baltimore, MD 21287, USA
* Corresponding author.
E-mail address: phg.jhu@me.com (P. Gailloud).

Neuroimag Clin N Am 19 (2009) 169–179
doi:10.1016/j.nic.2009.02.001

taken from several primitive arterial systems. A few basic embryonic concepts are introduced to clarify the type of variations and collateral pathways existing in the orbital region. The following summary is based on works published by Padget[4] and by Maillot and colleagues.[5]

Early in the fetal life, the blood supply to the eye and optic nerve is provided by two primitive OAs. The primitive dorsal OA (PrDOA) appears first in the 4-mm embryo, followed by the primitive ventral ophthalmic artery (PrVOA) in the 9-mm embryo. The PrVOA is a branch of the cranial division of the internal carotid artery (ICA) (future anterior and middle cerebral arteries), whereas the PrDOA originates from the intracranial portion of the ICA, near its termination, distally to the final point of emergence of the adult OA. The PrDOA, therefore, is not a branch of the cavernous segment of the ICA; this misconception, disseminated in the literature, finds its source in a misreading of Padget's splendid work on the embryology of the cranial arteries.[4] In the 16- to 19-mm embryo, the temporociliary branch of the PrDOA and the nasociliary branch of the PrVOA fuse around the optic nerve, the PrDOA becomes dominant, and the PrVOA starts regressing. Concomitantly, the PrDOA migrates from its initial point of origin to a more proximal location consistent with the origin of the adult OA. The blood supply to the connective apparatus surrounding the optic elements comes, alternatively, from the primitive orbital artery, a branch of the ramus superior of the stapedial artery (ie, the future middle meningeal artery [MMA]). These various embryonic OA components are illustrated in **Fig. 1**.

In order to reach its normal adult configuration, the OA establishes a connection with the primitive orbital artery and takes over most of the orbital blood supply. The proximal segment of the primitive orbital artery involutes to become an anastomosis between the anterior division of the MMA and the lacrimal artery. This anastomosis has classically received different names for its intraorbital and intracranial segments (ie, the recurrent meningeal branch of the lacrimal artery and the orbital branch of the anterior division of the MMA, respectively). This arterial network seems more complex than initially appreciated, however, and the existence of a double connection between the MMA and the lacrimal artery has been demonstrated by several investigators.[6,7] One connecting branch is short and straight; it crosses the foramen of Hyrtl (or cranio-orbital foramen) and takes the name, meningolacrimal artery. The other is long and tortuous; it passes through the superior orbital fissure (SOF) and takes the name, sphenoidal

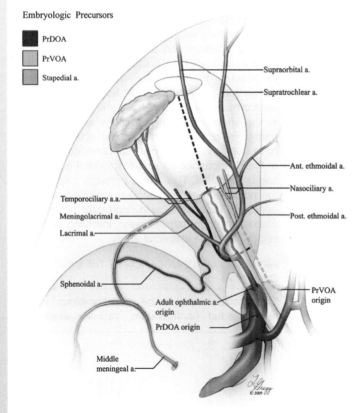

Embryologic Precursors

- PrDOA
- PrVOA
- Stapedial a.

Supraorbital a.
Supratrochlear a.
Ant. ethmoidal a.
Nasociliary a.
Post. ethmoidal a.
Temporociliary a.a.
Meningolacrimal a.
Lacrimal a.
Sphenoidal a.
Adult ophthalmic a. origin
PrDOA origin
PrVOA origin
Middle meningeal a.

Fig. 1. Schematic representation of the OA developmental anatomy and its adult derivatives. The dotted vascular segments normally are absent at the adult stage. The primitive OAs and their branches are shown in green (PrVOA) and purple (PrDOA). The segment of the hyaloid artery located within the vitreous humor starts involuting at approximately the 10th week of gestation (dotted purple), whereas its proximal segment becomes the adult central retinal artery. The structures shown in orange are derivatives of the stapedial artery (primitive orbital artery). The sphenoidal artery (red) is a late-appearing neomorph. (*Courtesy of* L. Gregg, Baltimore, MD; with permission. Copyright © Lydia Gregg 2009.)

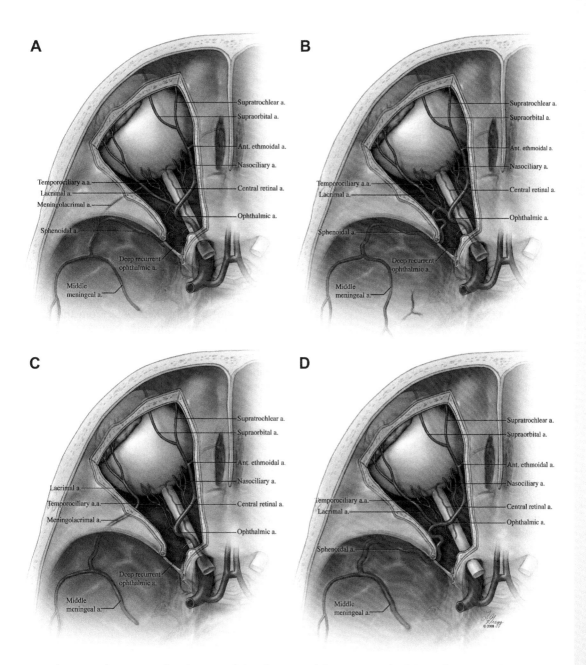

Fig. 2. The OA and its principal variants involving the MMA. (*A*) In its normal adult configuration, the OA originates from the ICA immediately after its passage through the dural ring and enters the orbital cavity through the optic canal. Connections with the MMA are established via the meningolacrimal artery through the foramen of Hyrtl and via the sphenoidal artery through the lateral aspect of the SOF. The meningolacrimal artery, short and straight, is the true vestige of the anterior ramus of the stapedial artery. The sphenoidal artery, long and tortuous, is a neomorph present only in hominids. The deep recurrent OA stems from the first part of the OA and courses backward through the medial aspect of the SOF to connect with the inferior-lateral trunk of the ICA. (*B*) The MMA can originate from the OA. The connection between the lacrimal artery and the MMA is believed to rely on the sphenoidal artery (as illustrated), although the meningolacrimal also could be involved. (*C*) The OA can originate from the MMA via the sphenoidal artery or via the meningolacrimal artery. In the latter instance (as illustrated), the abnormal OA has a relatively straight course and it penetrates the orbital cavity through the foramen of Hyrtl. The connection to the lacrimal artery is distal, a factor possibly explaining why, in this configuration, the OA tends to supply the orbit only partially, generally through the lacrimal artery. (*D*) When the sphenoidal artery is involved, the abnormal OA has a more tortuous course, enters the orbit via the lateral aspect of the SOF, and establishes a more proximal connection with the lacrimal artery. The authors believe that the potential for the abnormal OA to supply the entire orbital content, including the optic apparatus, is higher in this configuration (as illustrated). (*Courtesy of* L. Gregg, Baltimore, MD; with permission. Copyright © Lydia Gregg 2009.)

artery.[7] It remains uncertain if only one or both branches are derived from the stapedial artery (**Fig.** 2A). A recent review of available phylogenetic and ontogenetic data seems to indicate that the meningolacrimal artery is the true vestige of the stapedial artery, whereas the sphenoidal artery is a neomorph that appears late in the ontogenic development and seems restricted to hominids (man and orangutans).[8] Variations in the mode of connection of these various arteries and in their regression patterns are at the origin of the principal variants of the orbital supply and of several related dangerous collaterals. These variants (discussed later) include the origin of a part or of the whole MMA from the OA (see **Fig.** 2B) and the origin of the OA or one of its branches from the MMA (**Fig.** 2C, D).

Anatomy

The ophthalmic artery and its branches
The nomenclature used in this section is based, whenever possible, on the 1998 edition of *Terminologia Anatomica*.[9] The OA (arteria ophthalmica) is the first major branch of the ICA. As the site of origin of the OA usually is located at or close to the superior dural ring, it often is used as a point of demarcation between the intra- and extradural segments of the ICA. This landmark is somewhat imprecise: whereas the OA generally branches off the ICA immediately after the latter has pierced the roof of the cavernous sinus, in most cases within the subdural space,[10] this site of origin can vary proximally from the cavernous sinus up distally to the ICA bifurcation. Rarely, the OA can originate within the two layers of the dural roof.[10] The intracranial segment of the OA has a short

course within the subdural space before it enters the optic canal. It is followed by the intracanalicular portion of the OA, which often can be identified by a slight decrease of its caliber throughout the length of the optic canal.[11] The OA courses below the optic nerve in its intracranial and intracanalicular segments.[11] The intraorbital segment of the OA has been divided in three parts by Hayreh and Dass.[12] As it penetrates the orbital cavity through the common anular ring (tendon of Zinn), the OA first lies inferiorly and laterally to the optic nerve (first part). It then loops above (82.6%) or below (17.4%) the nerve to reach its superior-medial aspect (second part). This semicircular course around the nerve is a vestige of the connection between the nasociliary and temporociliary branches of the primitive OAs. From that point, the OA aims anteriorly and medially toward the orbital wall (third part), ending at the superior-medial aspect of the orbital opening, although its caliber often is already significantly reduced distal to the take off of the anterior ethmoidal artery.[12]

A complete description of the branches of the OA is beyond the scope of this article. For more detailed reference, readers are directed to the classic work of Hayreh.[13] It is convenient to classify the branches of the OA according to their topography.[13] The ocular group, which includes the branches supplying the optic apparatus (central retinal, ciliary, and collateral arteries), are not discussed further. The lacrimal and muscular arteries remain within the confine of the orbital cavity and constitute the orbital group, along with various smaller branches supplying the surrounding connective structures. Finally, the extra-orbital group includes branches that exit the orbital cavity, such as the posterior and

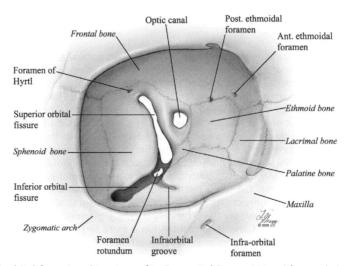

Fig. 3. The principal orbital foramina. (*Courtesy of* L. Gregg, Baltimore, MD; with permission. Copyright © Lydia Gregg 2009.)

anterior ethmoidal, the medial palpebral, the dorsal nasal, and the supratrochlear arteries. Several branches of the lacrimal artery are part of this group, including the sphenoidal and meningolacrimal arteries. The first part of the OA also provides two small recurrent arteries. One of them exits the orbit through the medial aspect of the SOF and establishes a connection with the inferior-lateral trunk of the cavernous ICA (C4 segment). This branch, known as the deep recurrent OA, seems to be a stable feature of the OA anatomy[14] and plays a significant role in several OA variations. The second recurrent branch, the superficial recurrent OA, seems less constant and represents one of the possible origins of the marginal tentorial artery.[14]

The orbital foramina

A brief description of some of the various foramina connecting the orbital cavity to its surroundings helps understand most of the variants and anastomoses (discussed later). These principal foramina are illustrated in **Fig. 3.**

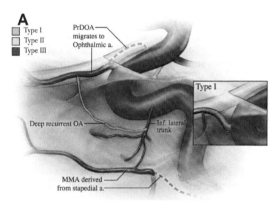

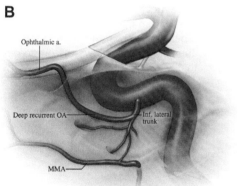

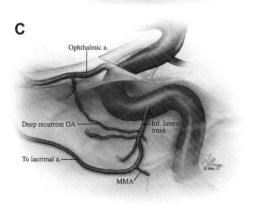

Fig. 4. Cavernous origin of the OA types I, II, and III. (*A*) This illustration depicts the embryonic precursors of the OA and their role in several variants of the OA origin. The green dotted line represents the primary origin of the PrDOA. A true persistence of the fetal configuration results in an OA arising from the ICA at the level of the posterior communicating artery. The deep recurrent OA is shown in yellow. The stapedial artery and a persistent connection with the inferior lateral trunk of the ICA are shown in purple, whereas its involuted origin from the petrous ICA is shown in orange. The inset illustrates a cavernous OA type I. In this variant, the OA originates from the ICA close to the dural ring; it then assumes a sharp upward curve to enter the optic canal. From that point on, a cavernous OA type I has the course and distribution of a normal OA. (*B*) In a cavernous OA type II, the OA originates from the horizontal segment of the cavernous ICA; it corresponds to the deep recurrent OA, a branch of the inferior-lateral trunk. The abnormal OA, therefore, penetrates the orbit via the medial aspect of the SOF and continues as the first part of the OA. This proximal connection implies that cavernous OA type II supply the entire ophthalmic distribution, including the optic apparatus. (*C*) A cavernous OA type III also originates from the horizontal segment of the ICA, but in this case, the connection is established with the stapedial artery (or, at the adult stage, with the MMA). A cavernous OA type III has the course and distribution of the anterior ramus of the stapedial artery, in a way that is similar to the variants presented in **Fig. 1.** It enters the orbital cavity via the foramen of Hyrtl if it involves the meningolacrimal artery or via the lateral aspect of the SOF if it involves the sphenoidal artery. (*Courtesy of* L. Gregg, Baltimore, MD; with permission. Copyright © Lydia Gregg 2009.)

1. The optic canal (canalis opticus) is contained within the base of the lesser wing of the sphenoid bone. The optic nerve and the OA enter the orbital cavity through the optic canal. In rare instances, the OA can penetrate a separate osseous canal that joins the optic canal near its orbital end.[10]

2. The SOF (fissura orbitalis superior) is delimited superiorly by the lesser wing and inferiorly by the greater wing of the sphenoid bone. It is pear-shaped, with a wide medial-inferior base and a narrow lateral-superior tail. The two edges of the fissure usually remain separate until they reach the frontal bone. A small foramen, the ophthalmomeningeal foramen of Hyrtl (or cranio-orbital foramen), can be seen laterally to the SOF, sometimes close enough to be confluent with its lateral extremity.[8] When present, this foramen gives way to an anastomosis between the lacrimal artery and the MMA, the meningolacrimal artery, which is believed to represent the vestige of the superior ramus of the stapedial artery (ie, the primitive orbital artery). A second anastomosis between the lacrimal artery and the MMA, the sphenoidal artery (often confusingly identified as the recurrent meningeal branch of the lacrimal artery), is believed to be a neomorph present only in some hominids, including man. The sphenoidal artery passes through the lateral aspect of the SOF[15] and is involved in several major OA variants. The middle portion of the SOF contains the superior ophthalmic vein, whereas the medial portion gives way to the inferior ophthalmic vein. The deep recurrent OA also passes through the medial portion of the SOF, crossing the tendon of Zinn.[14]

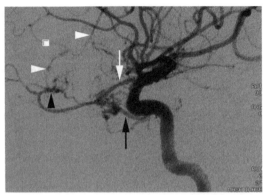

Fig. 6. Right ICA angiogram (lateral projection) in a 17-year-old boy who had orbital fibrous dysplasia. The inferior lateral trunk participates in the vascularization of the osseous pathology via several branches including a prominent deep recurrent OA (*black arrow*). The latter can be followed from the inferior-lateral trunk up to its connection with the first part of an OA of normal origin (*white arrow*). Note that in this patient, the lacrimal artery (*black arrowhead*) branches off the MMA (*white arrowheads*). (*Courtesy of* L. Gregg, Baltimore, MD; with permission. Copyright © Lydia Gregg 2009.)

3. The inferior orbital fissure (IOF) (fissura orbitalis inferior) connects the orbital cavity with the infratemporal fossa and, through the latter, with the more medially located pterygopalatine fossa. Coming from the pterygopalatine fossa, the infraorbital artery (with its vein) enters the orbit via the IOF. It first follows the infraorbital groove that stems anteriorly from the IOF

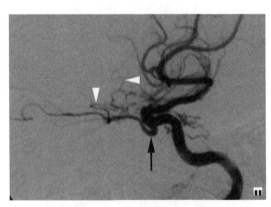

Fig. 7. Right ICA angiogram, lateral projection, showing a cavernous OA type II. The OA originates from the horizontal segment of the cavernous ICA (*black arrow*) and penetrates the orbital cavity through the medial aspect of the SOF to continue as the first segment of the OA, supplying the entire OA distribution. In this case, the lacrimal artery provides the MMA (*white arrowheads*). (*Courtesy of* L. Gregg, Baltimore, MD; with permission. Copyright © Lydia Gregg 2009.)

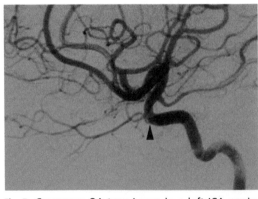

Fig. 5. Cavernous OA type I seen in a left ICA angiogram, lateral projection. The OA originates from the ICA close to the dural ring (*black arrowhead*) and curves sharply upwards to enter the optic canal. (*Courtesy of* L. Gregg, Baltimore, MD; with permission. Copyright © Lydia Gregg 2009.)

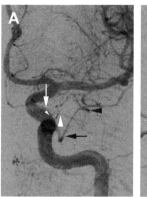
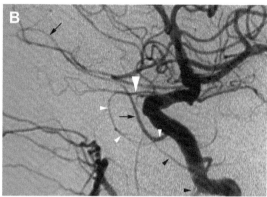

Fig. 8. Cavernous OA type III seen on a left common carotid angiogram. (A) In this anteroposterior projection, a small OA of normal origin (*white arrow*) enters the orbital cavity through the optic canal (*white arrowhead*) to supply the optic apparatus. A cavernous OA type III (*black arrow*) originates from the cavernous ICA and enters the orbit through the foramen of Hyrtl (*black arrowhead*). This branch supplies the orbital content other than the optic apparatus. This configuration reproduces the embryonic stage during which the orbital vascularization is shared between the primitive orbital artery (from the stapedial artery) and the PrDOA. In addition, a deep recurrent OA is partially seen projecting over the distal ICA (*small white arrowhead*). (B) The lateral oblique projection confirms the presence of a "normal" OA supplying the optic apparatus (*white arrowhead*) in addition to a cavernous OA type III (*black arrows*). The course of the deep recurrent OA is shown by the small white arrowheads back to its connection with the inferior-lateral trunk. Note the presence of a diminutive MMA (*black arrowheads*) connecting to the proximal segment of the cavernous OA type III, confirming the homology of the latter with the anterior ramus of the stapedial artery. (*Courtesy of* L. Gregg, Baltimore, MD; with permission. Copyright © Lydia Gregg 2009.)

(sulcus infraorbitalis), then courses within the infraorbital canal (canalis infraorbitalis) and exits the orbit through the infraorbital foramen (foramen infraorbitale).

4. The anterior ethmoidal foramen (foramen ethmoidale anterius) and the posterior ethmoidal foramen (foramen ethmoidale posterius) contain the anterior and posterior ethmoidal arteries, respectively. The anterior ethmoidal artery provides an important meningeal branch, the anterior meningeal artery, which enters the cranial cavity via the ethmoidal foramen of the cribriform plate.

Anatomic Variants and Dangerous Collaterals

Cavernous origin of the ophthalmic artery

Three types of cavernous origin of the OA can be differentiated (Fig. 4A–C). In type I, the origin of the OA lies close to the dural ring, and the vessel

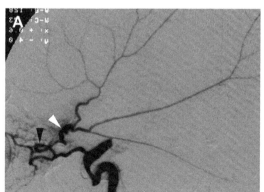
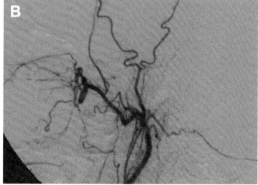

Fig. 9. OA origin of the MMA. (A) Angiography of the left ICA, lateral projection, in a patient who had embolic occlusion of the distal ICA (the image has been flipped horizontally for consistency with other figures). The lacrimal artery (*black arrowhead*) is providing the MMA. Note the tortuous appearance of the arterial segment running between the lacrimal artery and the MMA (*white arrowhead*), consistent with the course of the sphenoidal artery. (B) Angiography of the left ECA, lateral projection, confirming the absence of a normal MMA from the maxillary artery. (*Courtesy of* L. Gregg, Baltimore, MD; with permission. Copyright © Lydia Gregg 2009.)

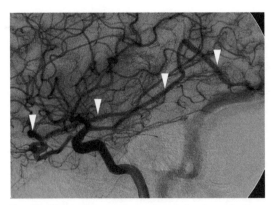

Fig. 10. Right ICA angiography, lateral projection, showing a prominent MMA (*white arrowheads*) originating from the lacrimal artery and feeding a right transverse sinus DAVF. (*Courtesy of* L. Gregg, Baltimore, MD; with permission. Copyright © Lydia Gregg 2009.)

OA arises more proximally from the ICA (C3 or C4 segment) and penetrates into the orbit via the medial aspect of the SOF (type II) or through its lateral aspect or the foramen of Hyrtl (type III). The abnormal vessel can be the only detectable OA (generally type II) or it can partially supply the orbit, generally providing only the lacrimal artery (type III). In the latter instance, the cavernous OA is associated with a second OA, which usually has a normal adult origin. The authors believe that types II and III have different embryonic origins. Type II seems to correspond to the deep recurrent OA, a branch of the inferior lateral trunk that normally penetrates the orbit via the medial aspect of the SOF and the tendon of Zinn (Fig. 6). Because the deep recurrent OA is connected with the first part of the OA, a cavernous OA type II generally takes over the supply of the entire orbital content (Fig. 7). Cavernous OAs type III represent, in the authors' opinion, a true vestige of the stapedial artery, more precisely of the proximal segment of the primitive orbital artery, and of its connection with the C4 segment of the ICA, an idea put forward by Maillot and coworkers.[5] This developmental anatomy is consistent with the observation that a cavernous OA type III often is associated with a small or absent ipsilateral MMA and that it enters the orbit crossing the lateral aspect of the SOF or the foramen of Hyrtl (Fig. 8). Cavernous OAs type III and variants in which the OA originates from the MMA, therefore, are similar. Both have the same distal anatomy and vary only by their site of origin (ie, from the ICA for the former [connection of the stapedial artery with the ICA] and from the MMA

assumes a sharp upward curve to enter the optic canal (Fig. 5). In this variant, the proximal segment of the OA derives from the PrDOA, as it is the case in the normal adult configuration. The proximal origin of the OA could be related to an exaggerated caudal migration of the PrDOA.[5]

Types II and III often are described as persistent dorsal OAs, although these variants are better labeled as cavernous origins of the OA, because they do not represent the persistence of the PrDOA. The PrDOA is not a branch of the cavernous segment of the ICA.[4] The exceptional adult persistence of the origin of the PrDOA results in an OA coming from the ICA distally to its expected adult position. In types II and III, the

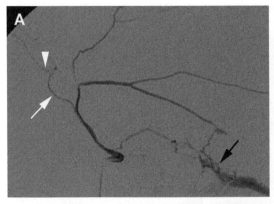

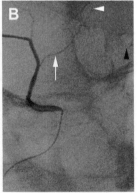

Fig. 11. Right external carotid artery angiography in a case of transverse sinus DAVF. (*A*) The lateral projection shows the meningolacrimal artery (anterior ramus of the stapedial artery) (*white arrow*) continuing within the orbital cavity as the lacrimal artery (*white arrowhead*). Note the straight course of the connecting segment consistent with the anatomy of the meningolacrimal artery. The MMA is feeding a transverse sinus DAVF (*black arrow*). (*B*) The anteroposterior projection confirms the passage of the connecting segment of the meningolacrimal artery (*white arrow*) through the foramen of Hyrtl or the lateral end of the SOF (*whiter arrowhead*), at distance from the optic canal (*black arrowhead*). (*Courtesy of* L. Gregg, Baltimore, MD; with permission. Copyright © Lydia Gregg 2009.)

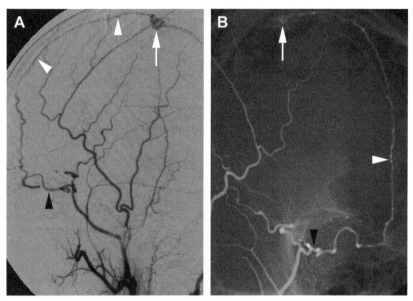

Fig. 12. Right external carotid artery angiography in a case of transverse sinus DAVF. (A) The lateral view shows a prominent OA coming from the MMA (black arrowhead) and feeding a superior sagittal sinus DAVF (white arrow) via the anterior meningeal artery (a branch of the anterior ethmoidal artery) (white arrowheads). Note the tortuous appearance of the proximal segment of the OA (sphenoidal type). (B) The right anterior oblique view shows the tortuous path followed by the proximal segment of the OA (black arrowhead), consistent with the anatomy of a sphenoidal artery, and its medial course across the orbital cavity ending near the anterior ethmoidal foramen, through which it provides a large branch vascularizing the DAVF (white arrow). (Courtesy of L. Gregg, Baltimore, MD; with permission. Copyright © Lydia Gregg 2009.)

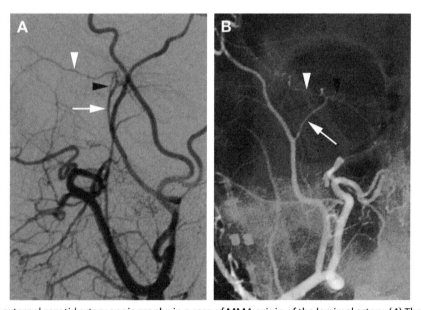

Fig. 13. Right external carotid artery angiography in a case of MMA origin of the lacrimal artery. (A) The lateral view shows the smooth continuation of the anterior branch of the MMA (white arrow) into the lacrimal artery (white arrowhead), typical of the meningolacrimal configuration. A second, more tortuous and medially oriented branch is observed (black arrowhead). (B) The anteroposterior projection confirms the presence of a meningolacrimal artery entering the orbital cavity laterally and continuing as the lacrimal artery (white arrowhead). The second branch has a medial course and the typical tortuosity of a sphenoidal artery (black arrowhead). The risk linked to the presence of a dangerous connection with branches supplying the optic apparatus through the sphenoidal artery is higher in this configuration than in cases where the meningolacrimal artery is isolated and provides only the lacrimal artery. The white arrow indicates the anterior branch of the MMA. (Courtesy of L. Gregg, Baltimore, MD; with permission. Copyright © Lydia Gregg 2009.)

for the latter [connection of the stapedial artery with the ECA]). The connection of cavernous OAs type III with the orbital arterial system is established at the level of the lacrimal artery via a meningolacrimal artery or a sphenoidal artery. As discussed later, the extent of orbital supply provided by the variant may depend in part on which of these two connections is involved.

Ophthalmic origin of the middle meningeal artery

The MMA may originate partially or completely from the lacrimal artery. Two arterial segments can explain such a variation. The MMA can result from the persistence of the segment of stapedial artery corresponding to the primitive orbital artery (later known as the meningolacrimal artery) and exit the orbit via the foramen of Hyrtl. Alternatively, the connection can involve an arterial segment believed to be a late-acquired neomorph, the sphenoidal artery, and exit the orbit via the lateral aspect the SOF. In both instances, the foramen spinosum is hypoplastic or absent. It has been proposed that a MMA arising from the OA is derived more often from a sphenoidal artery;[8]

this seems consistent with the observation that, in such a variant, the proximal segment of the MMA usually has a tortuous course, a typical feature of the sphenoidal artery (Fig. 9).

A MMA arising from the OA may be involved in various pathologic processes and can in particular participate in the vascularization of meningeal lesions, such as a meningioma or a dural arteriovenous fistula (DAVF) (Fig. 10).

Middle meningeal origin of the ophthalmic artery

The MMA can partially or completely provide blood supply to the orbital content. Again, two pathways may link the MMA to the lacrimal artery. The original connection of the primitive orbital artery with the intraorbital network can remain patent and prominent. In this case, the MMA generally provides only the lacrimal artery via a short and straight connection through the foramen of Hyrtl. This anatomy is consistent with the typical appearance of the meningolacrimal artery and with its relatively distal connection with the lacrimal artery (Fig. 11). The second pathway involves the sphenoidal artery. In this

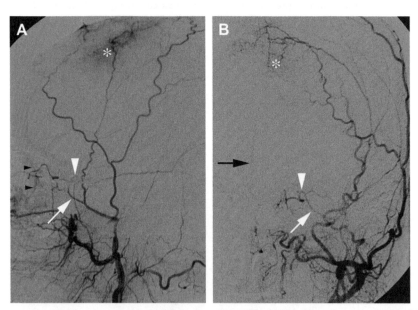

Fig. 14. Left external carotid artery angiography in a patient who had a frontal meningioma. (A) The lateral projection shows a prominent OA arising from the anterior division of the MMA (*white arrow*). Note the tortuous course of the OA as it enters the orbital cavity, an appearance consistent with a sphenoidal type (*white arrowhead*). The presence of a choroid blush (*black arrowheads*) confirms the participation of the variant to the blood supply of the optic apparatus. The white asterisk indicates the tumoral blush of the meningioma. (B) The anteroposterior projection confirms the sinuous medial trajectory of the extraorbital segment of the OA (sphenoidal type) (*white arrowhead*) and the extent of its intraorbital supply, including a small lacrimal artery traveling laterally and a larger main stem aiming medially toward the anterior ethmoidal foramen. The anterior meningeal branch of the anterior ethmoidal artery (*black arrow*) is involved in the supply of the meningioma (*asterisk*). The *white arrow* indicates the anterior division of the MMA. (*Courtesy of* L. Gregg, Baltimore, MD; with permission. Copyright © Lydia Gregg 2009.)

case, the connection often shows significant tortuosity as the connecting segment travels medially, and the MMA tends to provide a larger part of the orbital supply, sometimes its entirety. This is in keeping with the appearance of the sphenoidal artery and its relatively proximal connection with the lacrimal artery (**Fig. 12**). The meningolacrimal and sphenoidal arteries can at times be observed simultaneously (**Fig. 13**).

Although all of these OA variations need to be considered dangerous anastomoses, the possibility that the MMA supplies important optic structures (in particular via the central retinal artery) is higher for variants of the sphenoidal type than for those of the meningolacrimal type, in particular when the latter is associated with a well-defined second OA. Transarterial embolization in the MMA territory must be considered high risk and attempted only after careful evaluation of the procedural risks and benefits whenever the MMA provides the main trunk of the OA and likely supplies the optic apparatus (eg, in the sphenoidal type of the variation, with or without an angiographically detectable choroid blush) (**Fig. 14**).

An OA originating from the MMA may be involved in various neurovascular conditions. Through the anterior ethmoidal artery and its anterior meningeal branch, it can supply blood to a meningioma or a DAVF (see **Figs. 11** and **14**). A MMA that vascularizes the optic apparatus may be involved in a central retinal artery occlusion and become the target vessel for intra-arterial thrombolysis (P. Gailloud, MD, and colleagues, unpublished data, 2007).

SUMMARY

Three types of cavernous origins of the OA can be distinguished. In a cavernous OA type I, the OA has an extradural origin but a normal course through the optic canal and a normal intraorbital branching pattern. A cavernous OA type II derives from the deep recurrent OA. As the latter branch is normally connected to the first part of the OA, type II generally supplies the entire ophthalmic territory. Embolization of a cavernous OA type II, therefore, requires the same risk-benefit analysis as does embolization in the distribution of a normal OA. Cavernous OA type III involves the anterior ramus of the stapedial artery and, except for its origin from the ICA, is similar to variants in which the OA comes from the MMA. In both instances, the connection with the ophthalmic circulation is established more distally, at the level of the lacrimal artery, via a meningolacrimal artery (through the foramen of Hyrtl) or via a sphenoidal artery (through the lateral aspect of the SOF).

Although they still must be considered high-risk vessels for embolization, a cavernous OA type III or an OA coming from the MMA is less likely to be involved in the vascularization of the optic apparatus, particularly when they are derived from the meningolacrimal artery (straight connection) or when a second OA coming from the ICA is detected. The same reasoning can be applied to OAs arising from the MMA.

REFERENCES

1. Merland JJ, Djindjian R, Bories J. Superselective arteriography of the branches of the external carotid artery. Recent findings concerning the exo- and endocranial base of the skull. Berlin. New York: Springer-Verlag; 1975.
2. Lasjaunias PL, Berenstein A. Craniofacial and upper cervical arteries: functional, clinical, and angiographic aspects. Baltimore (MD): Williams & Wilkins; 1981.
3. Marinkovic S, Gibo A, Brigante L, et al. Arteries of the brain and spinal cord. Anatomic features and clinical significance. Avellino (Italy): De Angelis; 1997.
4. Padget DH. The development of cranial arteries in the human embryo. Contrib Embryol 1948;32:205–61.
5. Maillot C, Froelich S, Kehrli P. [Ophthalmic artery, optic nerve and meninges: reciprocal relations]. J Neuroradiol 2000;27:93–100.
6. Moret J, Lasjaunias P, Theron J, et al. The middle meningeal artery. Its contribution to the vascularisation of the orbit. J Neuroradiol 1977;4:225–48.
7. Lasjaunias P, Vignaud J, Hasso AN. Maxillary artery blood supply to the orbit: normal and pathological aspects. Neuroradiology 1975;9:87–97.
8. Diamond MK. Homologies of the meningeal-orbital arteries of humans: a reappraisal. J Anat 1991;178:223–41.
9. Federative Committee on Anatomical Terminology. Terminologia anatomica: international anatomical terminology. Stuttgart (NY): Thieme; 1998.
10. Hayreh SS, Dass R. The ophthalmic artery: I. Origin and intra-cranial and intra-canalicular course. Br J Ophthalmol 1962;46:65–98.
11. Dilenge D. L' angiographie par soustraction de l'artère ophtalmique et de ses branches. Paris: Masson; 1965 [in French].
12. Hayreh SS, Dass R. The ophthalmic artery: II. Intra-orbital course. Br J Ophthalmol 1962;46:165–85.
13. Hayreh SS. The ophthalmic artery: III. Branches. Br J Ophthalmol 1962;46:212–47.
14. Lasjaunias P, Brismar J, Moret J, et al. Recurrent cavernous branches of the ophthalmic artery. Acta Radiol Diagn (Stockh) 1978;19:553–60.
15. Martins C, Yasuda A, Campero A, et al. Microsurgical anatomy of the dural arteries. Neurosurgery 2005;56:211–51 [discussion: 51].

Embolization of Vascular Tumors of the Head and Neck

Joseph J. Gemmete, MD[a],*, Sameer A. Ansari, MD, PhD[b],
Jonathan McHugh, MD[c], Dheeraj Gandhi, MD[d]

KEYWORDS

- Head and neck tumor • Preoperative tumor embolization
- Therapeutic embolization • Direct puncture

This article provides an overview of embolization of vascular tumors of the head and neck, with emphasis on recent advancements in endovascular techniques available for treatment. The authors first discuss the functional vascular anatomy and technical aspects of head and neck embolization. In the subsequent sections, they present a detailed discussion of the two most common head and neck tumors, juvenile nasopharyngeal angiofibromas (JNAs) and paragangliomas, which require embolization as an adjunct to surgery. Finally, the authors discuss their experiences at the University of Michigan.

FUNCTIONAL VASCULAR ANATOMY

An understanding of the anatomy of the external carotid artery (ECA) is essential for performing safe and effective embolization of vascular tumors of the head and neck because of the many anatomic variations, territorial anastomoses, and collateral supplies found in this region.[1] The anatomy of the ECA is variable and is best considered on a functional basis. In particular, for cases in which one artery is small, that area is then supplied by an enlarged neighboring branch. The blood supply to tumors of the head and neck is derived from regional vasculature and is provided by branches of the ECA with additional recruitment of the vertebral artery (VA), internal carotid artery (ICA), and thyrocervical or costocervical trunk, depending on the size and location of the tumor. Tumors adjacent to the brain may parasitize regional pial blood supply as they enlarge.

Prevention of serious complications requires knowledge and recognition of the territorial anastomoses. Anastomotic pathways exist between the ECA, ICA, VA, ophthalmic artery, ascending cervical artery, deep cervical artery, and spinal arteries, which are embryologic remnants from early fetal life. The most common dangerous anastomoses involve communications of the first- or second-order branches of the ECA (the ascending pharyngeal [APA], occipital [OA], middle meningeal [MMA], accessory meningeal [AMA], and distal internal maxillary arteries [IMA]) with the ICA or VA. Furthermore, the MMA, IMA, superficial temporal, and facial arteries can all anastomose with the ophthalmic artery.[2] These anastomoses may not be evident on an initial angiogram, but may reveal themselves as the changes in the regional blood flow occur during the embolization. Endovascular surgeons need to be familiar with these connections when embolizing tumors within any of these vascular territories to avoid inadvertent passage of the embolic material to the retina or the central nervous system. The ECA system provides collateral circulation for the ICA and is

a Division of Interventional Neuroradiology, Department of Radiology, University of Michigan Health System, 1500 E. Medical Center Dr., B1D330, Ann Arbor, MI 48109-0030, USA
b Departments of Radiology, Neurology, and Surgery, University of Chicago Medical Center, 5841 S. Maryland Avenue, MC-2026, Chicago, IL 60637, USA
c Department of Pathology, University of Michigan Health System, Ann Arbor, MI, USA
d Johns Hopkins University and Hospitals, Departments of Radiology, Neurology, and Neurosurgery, Division of Interventional Neuroradiology, 600 N Wolfe St/Radiology B-100, Baltimore, MD 21287, USA
* Corresponding author.
E-mail address: gemmete@umich.edu (J.J. Gemmete).

Neuroimag Clin N Am 19 (2009) 181–198
doi:10.1016/j.nic.2009.01.008

the primary blood supply to many of the cranial nerves. Palsies of cranial nerves V, VII, IX, X, XI, or XII may result from inappropriate embolization of the feeding branches to the vasa nervosum.[3] Selection of the correct embolic agent and, if required, provocative testing before embolization may help to avoid damage to the cranial nerves.[4,5]

TECHNICAL ASPECTS OF HEAD AND NECK TUMOR EMBOLIZATION

The tumors that require embolization in the head and neck most commonly include paragangliomas and JNAs. Other tumors that may require preoperative embolization include hypervascular metastases, schwannomas, rhabdomyosarcomas, extracranial meningiomas, esthesioneuroblastomas, neuroblastomas, endolymphatic sac tumors, and hemangiopericytomas.

The goal of tumor embolization is to selectively occlude the ECA feeders using intratumoral deposition of the embolic material.[6] The embolic agents commonly used include the following:

- polyvinyl alcohol
- trisacryl microspheres (Figs. 1–4)
- liquid n-butyl cyanoacrylate (n-BCA) Trufill (Cordis Neurovascular Inc., Miami Lakes, Florida) (see Fig. 3)
- ethyl-vinyl alcohol copolymer (EVOH) Onyx (ev3, Irvine, California) (see Figs. 1 and 4)
- gelfoam pledgets
- microcoils.

The embolization is ideally performed from 24 to 72 hours before the surgical resection to allow time for maximal thrombosis of the occluded vessels and prevent recanalization of the occluded arteries or formation of collateral arterial channels.[7,8] Preoperative embolization is cost-effective and tends to shorten operative time by reducing blood loss and the period of recovery.[9]

Treatment begins with first obtaining a detailed cerebral angiogram that includes selective injections of the common carotid artery, ICA, ECA, VA, and thyrocervical and costocervical trunks of the subclavian artery. A microcatheter is then advanced using fluoroscopic guidance into the artery supplying the tumor, and a microcatheter angiogram is performed to check for dangerous anastomoses between the ECA and ICA or vertebral arteries. The appropriate embolic agent is then injected using constant fluoroscopic monitoring, making sure to avoid reflux of embolic material and being vigilant for any dangerous anastomoses. If critical anastomoses are present, the anastomotic connection can be occluded using coils and then the particulate embolization

can be performed. Ideally, the embolic material is deposited at the arteriolar/capillary level. If there is arteriovenous shunting within the tumor, the particle size may need to be increased to prevent passage into the venous side. Proximal occlusion of the arterial feeders is inadequate because it allows arterial collateralization and may make surgical removal more difficult.

The authors prefer using trisacryl microspheres of 100 to 300 μm because these particles allow more distal penetration into the tumor bed and better devascularization.[10] However, one should always be aware of the possible risk for devascularizing the cranial nerves (the vasa nervosum are usually smaller than 60 μm) and the skin. In addition to potential central and peripheral nervous system damage, undesired embolization of normal external carotid territories can cause mucosal and tongue necrosis, laryngeal damage, and ocular damage. Smaller particles may also increase the risk for tumoral hemorrhage and swelling.[11] When embolizing the arterial pedicles that might also supply the cranial nerves (eg, the stylomastoid branch of the OA or the neuromeningeal trunk of the APA), the authors increase the particle size to from 300 to 500 μm. Similarly, the authors generally avoid liquid embolic agents (eg, n-BCA or EVOH), preferring to use a transarterial approach with particulate material, because liquid embolic agents can potentially occlude the arterial supply to the cranial nerves and may pass through the tiny anastomoses into the intracranial circulation.

Direct percutaneous puncture of tumors when using fluoroscopic, ultrasound, or CT guidance has also been described as a method to embolize a number of different tumors (see Figs. 1, and 4, 3). The method was initially reported for use in tumors in which conventional transarterial embolization was technically impossible because of the small size of the arterial feeders or involvement of branches arising from the ICA or VA feeding the tumor.[12] Examples include large tumors with supply from the ICA, VA, or ophthalmic artery for which devascularization from an intra-arterial approach using a microcatheter may not be possible or for which there may be significant risk for reflux of particles into the intracranial circulation or the retina. Excellent results obtained using this technique have extended its application to smaller and less complex tumors.[13] Direct and easy access to the vascular tumor bed that is not hampered by arterial tortuosity, the small size of the arterial feeders, atherosclerotic disease, or catheter-induced vasospasm is the main advantage of this technique.

Complete devascularization of the tumor can be obtained with decreased risk to the patient by using direct tumoral injection of n-BCA or

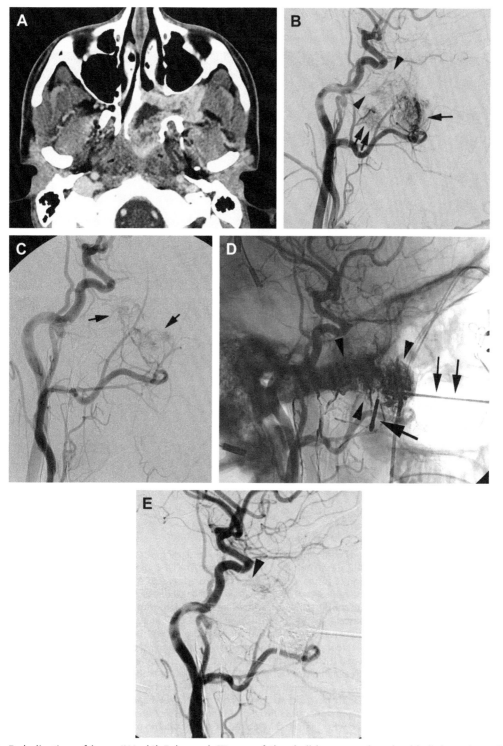

Fig. 1. Embolization of large JNA. (*A*) Enhanced CT scan of the skull base reveals a dumbbell-shaped, partially necrotic, and hypervascular mass on the left side. It originates in the region of the sphenopalatine foramen, which is also widened, and extends medially in the nasopharynx and laterally toward the infratemporal fossa. (*B*) Lateral angiogram of the left common carotid artery (CCA) demonstrates a hypervascular mass supplied by the IMA (*single arrow*), branches of the MMA (*double arrows*), and petrous and cavernous branches of the ICA (*arrowheads*). (*C*) Lateral CCA angiogram obtained after particle embolization of the distal IMA and branches of the MMA and APAs that supplied this neoplasm. Small amount of residual blush is present, supplied by tiny branches of the ECA and ICA (*arrows*). These branches are difficult to catheterize and embolize. (*D*) Transnasal (*double arrows*) and temporal approach (*single arrow*) was used for percutaneous access into the tumor bed, and Onyx was injected into the tumor bed using fluoroscopy (*arrowheads*). (*E*) Near-complete devascularization of the tumor is shown on this postembolization CCA angiogram. Note residual, minor opacification of the cavernous branch of the ICA (*arrowhead*).

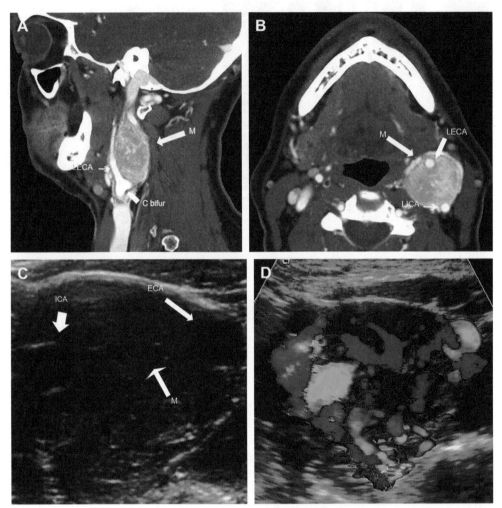

Fig. 2. Large, left-sided, carotid body paraganglioma (CBP), embolized using intra-arterial particulate material (250 cc total blood loss at resection). (*A*) Lateral multiplanar reformation of a CT angiogram shows a hypervascular mass (M) splaying the carotid bifurcation (C bifur). Left external carotid artery (LECA) is displaced anteriorly. (*B*) Axial, contrast-enhanced CT image of the neck shows a hypervascular mass (M) displacing the left internal carotid artery (LICA) posteriorly and the LECA anteriorly. (*C*, *D*) Ultrasound image (*C*) demonstrates a predominantly hypoechoic mass, which appears extremely vascular using color Doppler (*D*). (*E*) Lateral common carotid angiogram before embolization demonstrates this hypervascular mass (M) splaying the carotid bifurcation, a large area of blush, and multiple hypertrophied arterial feeders. (*F*) Lateral common carotid angiogram from late in the arterial phase reveals the extent of tumor blush and the complete margins of this hypervascular mass (M). (*G*) Lateral angiogram shows a microcatheter in a hypertrophied branch of the APA (*arrow*) before embolization. (*H*) Lateral, postemboli-zation angiogram demonstrates near-complete devascularization. (*I*) Gross pathology photograph shows circum-scribed paraganglioma (3.8 cm) with necrotic, whitish-yellow foci (*arrowheads*) associated with intravascular particles (*asterisks*) and surrounding peripheral viable (*tan*) tumor. (*J*) Viable paraganglioma (*left side*) and necrotic paraganglioma (*asterisk*) associated with a large, thin-walled vessel containing numerous particles (trisacryl micro-spheres, 100–300 μm, original magnification ×4). The particles are round, eosinophilic, and associated with fibrin and inflammatory cells (inset, original magnification ×20). ECA, external carotid; ICA, internal carotid artery; M, mass.

Onyx.[12,13] Onyx is a liquid embolic agent for pre-surgical embolization of cerebral arteriovenous malformations that has recently been approved by the US Food and Drug Administration. Onyx is a nonadhesive liquid embolic agent that is supplied in ready-to-use vials in a mixture with EVOH, dimethyl sulfoxide solvent (DMSO) and tantalum. Currently 6% (Onyx 18) and 8% (Onyx 34) EVOH concentrations (dissolved in DMSO) are available in the United States. Onyx is me-chanically occlusive but nonadherent to the vessel wall. Its nonadherent properties allow for a slow single injection of the embolic agent over a long period of time. During direct injection,

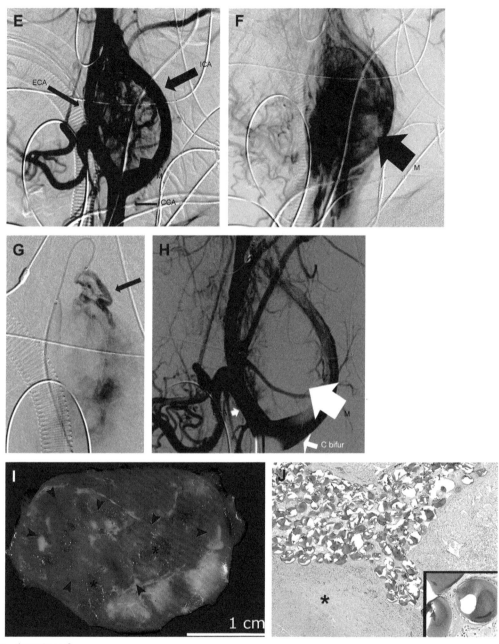

Fig. 2. (*continued*)

if unfavorable filling of the normal vascular structures occurs, the injection can be stopped and resumed after 30 seconds to 2 minutes. Solidification will occur in the embolized portion of the tumor. The injection can then be restarted, with Onyx taking the path of least resistance and filling another portion of the tumor. As the result of its properties, Onyx may potentially allow for a more controlled injection with better penetration into the tumor bed compared with n-BCA (see **Figs. 3** and **4**). Another benefit is that it advances in a single column, thus reducing the risk for involuntary venous migration.

The authors perform percutaneous injection of n-BCA or Onyx by placing an 18-gauge, short guiding needle into the tumor using fluoroscopic, ultrasound, or CT guidance and then coaxially introducing a 20-gauge spinal needle. After the needle is correctly located within the vascular bed of the tumor, a constant reflux of blood is observed. Contrast agent is injected through the needle and a tumorgram is obtained to assess

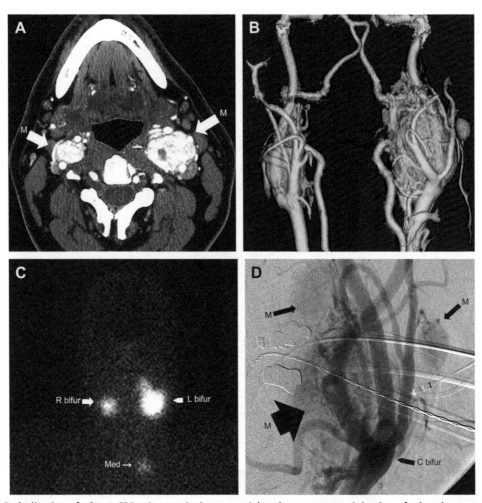

Fig. 3. Embolization of a large CBP using particulate material and percutaneous injection of n-butyl cyanoacrylate (n-BCA) (loss of <50 cc of blood at resection). Given the larger size and more rapid growth of the left CBP, its resection was planned first. (*A*) Axial, contrast-enhanced CT image of the neck shows bilateral hypervascular masses (M) consistent with CBPs at the carotid bifurcation. (*B*) Volume-rendered, three-dimensional reformat again demonstrates the masses at the carotid bifurcation bilaterally. (*C*) [111]indium-octreotide scan reveals increased radiotracer uptake at the carotid bifurcation bilaterally (R bifur, L bifur) and within the mediastinum (Med). (*D, E*) Frontal (*D*) and lateral (*E*) left common carotid angiograms demonstrate at least three hypervascular masses (M) in the region of the carotid bifurcation (C bifur). (*F*) Lateral, external carotid angiogram demonstrates filling of a hypervascular mass (M) from the occipital artery (OC) and a hypertrophied odontoid arcade (OD) off the ascending pharyngeal artery (APA). (*G*) Contrast injection through a needle (N) placed within the hypervascular mass (M) demonstrates filling of the internal tumor architecture. n-BCA glue cast (G) within the tumor from an injection of glue using a different needle (tumorgram, direct injection of contrast into the tumor). (*H, I*) Postembolization frontal (*H*) and lateral (*I*) left common carotid angiograms demonstrate complete devascularization of the mass after injection of from 100- to 300-μm particles and n-BCA (G). (*J*) Photomicrograph of a viable paraganglioma associated with large, thin-walled vessels (*white areas*) containing n-BCA and smaller vessels containing particles (original magnification ×4). The glue has mostly been dissolved out using tissue processing, but thin strands of fibrin remain, outlining where the n-BCA once was (inset, original magnification ×20). M, mass; N, needle.

for arterial reflux, venous drainage, potential for extravasation, and to determine which vascular compartment of the tumor will be filled with n-BCA or Onyx. The injection of the embolic agent is then performed using negative roadmapping. The procedure is stopped after complete devascularization is achieved, as determined by nonvisualization of intratumoral flow, or if the risk for potential arterial reflux into the intracranial circulation is considered to be high.

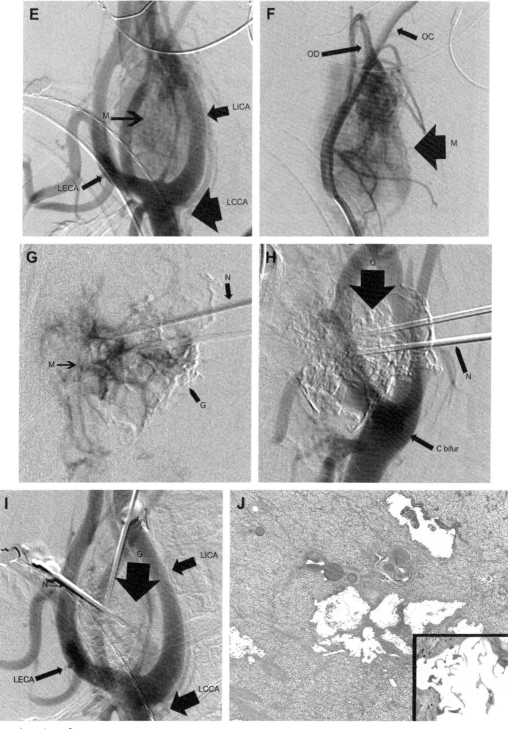

Fig. 3. (*continued*)

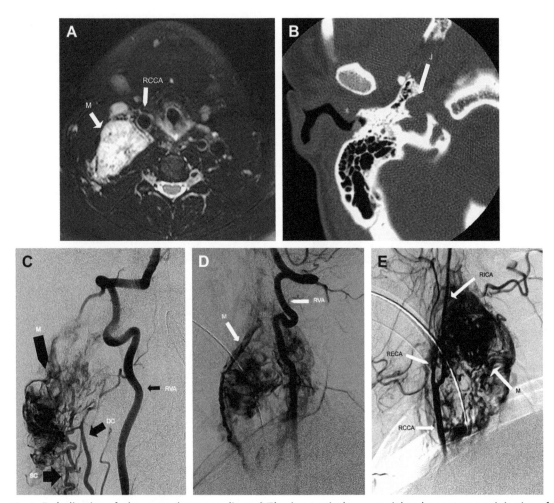

Fig. 4. Embolization of a large vagal paraganglioma (VP) using particulate material and percutaneous injection of Onyx (loss of <50 cc of blood at resection). (*A*) Axial, fat-saturated, T2-weighted MR image demonstrates a large mass within the neck (M). Note several flow voids within the tumor. RCCA, right common carotid artery. (*B*) Axial CT scan of the skull base with bone windows demonstrates a normal jugular bulb (J). (*C, D*) Frontal (*C*) and lateral (*D*) right subclavian arteriograms demonstrate a large hypervascular mass (M) with supply off the deep cervical (DC), superficial cervical (SC), and right vertebral arteries (RVA). (*E*) Lateral right common carotid arteriogram revealing an extremely vascular mass (M) located posteriorly in the carotid sheath. It displaces the right external carotid artery (RECA) and right internal carotid artery (RICA) anteriorly. (*F*) Lateral selective microcatheter angiogram of the occipital artery before particle embolization displays filling of the tumor vessels in this mass (M). (*G, H*) Lateral right subclavian arteriogram (*G*) and common carotid angiogram (*H*) after particulate and coil embolization of the arterial feeders from the right external carotid artery using trisacryl microspheres from 100 to 300 μm demonstrates residual filling of the mass (M). (*I*) Frontal contrast injection through the needle into the tumor, tumor gram (N) demonstrates opacification of the internal vascular architecture of the mass (M). (*J*) Frontal spot radiograph demonstrates the Onyx (O) cast with the mass. (*K*) Frontal right subclavian arteriogram demonstrates near-complete devascularization of the hypervascular mass. (*L*). Lateral right common carotid arteriogram confirms near-complete devascularization. (*M*) Photomicrograph of the resected specimen reveals a viable paraganglioma associated with large, thin-walled vessels containing numerous particles (trisacryl microspheres) and Onyx (black) (original magnification ×4). The Onyx is composed of black granular material that is nonrefractile and is associated with fibrin and inflammatory cells (Inset, original magnification ×20). C, coils; N, needle.

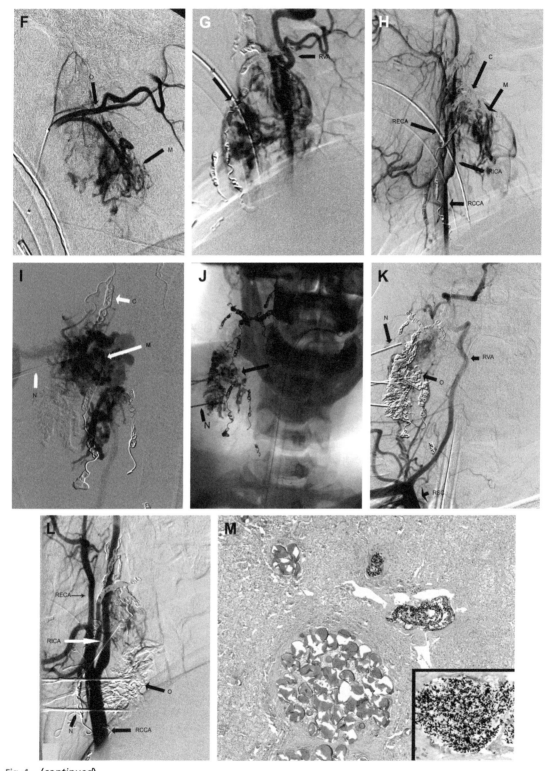

Fig. 4. (*continued*)

JUVENILE NASOPHARYNGEAL ANGIOFIBROMAS
Epidemiology

JNAs accounts for 0.5% of all head and neck tumors.[14,15] JNAs classically occur in adolescent males, with a peak incidence from 14 to 17 years of age.[16] JNAs are rare in patients older than 25 years of age. If the diagnosis of a JNA is made for a female patient, chromosomal analysis is recommended to exclude mosaicism.[17] No geographic or ethnic predilection has been reported.

Clinical Presentation

Patients generally present with nasal obstruction and recurrent epistaxis.[18] If drainage is impeded by the tumor, sinusitis or otitis may develop. Anosmia, proptosis, facial or temporal swelling, and extraocular muscle palsies may be seen, depending on the size and the direction of the tumor spread. On endoscopic examination, a lobulated, reddish-gray mass can be seen in the nasal cavity.[19]

Behavior and Location

JNAs are benign, fibrovascular tumors that are locally aggressive. Malignant conversion can occur; however, it is rare in tumors that have not been irradiated.[20,21] Spontaneous regression of the tumor has also been reported, but is again extremely rare.[22]

The tumors are thought to arise from the lateral margin of the posterior nasal cavity, adjacent to the sphenopalatine foramen. Large tumors are dumbbell-shaped or bi-lobed, with one portion of the tumor filling the nasopharynx and the other portion extending into the pterygopalatine fossa (see **Fig. 1**). These tumors can spread extensively along natural tissue planes. This spread may be anteriorly into the nasal cavity or medially toward the opposite nasal cavity (deforming and eroding the septum). Superiorly, the spread can occur into the sphenoid sinus, cavernous sinus, sella, and middle cranial fossa. Laterally, the tumor may spread into the pterygomaxillary and sphenopalatine fossae, bowing the posterior wall of the maxillary sinus and invading the infratemporal region. Occasionally, the great wing of the sphenoid bone may be eroded, exposing the dura of the middle cranial fossa.[16] The tumor generally does not invade bone, but does cause erosion and remodeling of bone.

Histology

On gross examination, the tumor is usually sessile, lobulated, rubbery, and red-pink to tan-gray in appearance. In rare cases, the tumor is polypoid or pedunculated. Nasopharyngeal angiofibroma is usually encapsulated and composed of vascular tissue and fibrous stroma with coarse or fine collagen fibers. Vessels are thin-walled, lack elastic fibers, have absent or incomplete smooth muscle, and under gross pathologic exam the vessels in the tumor appear stellate or staghorn in appearance to barely conspicuous because of stromal compression. Stromal cells have plump nuclei and tend to radiate around the vessels. There is an abundance of mast cells in the stroma and a lack of other inflammatory cells. Localized areas of myxomatous degeneration may be observed in the stroma.

When examined under an electron microscope, stromal cells can be identified as being mostly fibroblasts and show intensive immunostaining for vimentin. However, myofibroblasts may occur focally in connection with fibrotic areas and are characterized by the coexpression of vimentin and smooth muscle actin.[23]

Staging

A classification scheme for these tumors that was devised by Fisch[24] is summarized in **Table 1**. A widely used surgical staging system proposed by Radkowski and colleagues[25] for JNAs is given in **Table 2**.

Imaging

CT and MR imaging play a vital role in the assessment of these tumors. Axial and coronal CT images with bone windows best demonstrate the degree of bone remodeling and erosion. Pre- and postcontrast MR imaging best demonstrates the soft-tissue extent of the tumor and its vascularity. Differentiation between obstructed sinus secretions versus soft tissue mass from sinus invasion as well as intracranial extension is also best assessed using MR imaging.[26,27,28]

Angiography is usually performed in conjunction with preoperative embolization. Typical angiographic features include minimally dilated supplying arteries from the ECA and ICA, and an early-appearing, intense, but somewhat inhomogenous vascular blush that persists until late in the venous phase (see **Fig. 1**). Draining veins appear late in the angiogram, and arteriovenous shunting can be seen with these tumors. The lesion is generally supplied by branches of the IMA (the sphenopalatine and descending palatine branches), the anterior division of the APA, and the AMA. As the tumor grows, there is recruitment of other supply sources, including branches of the facial artery (ascending palatine artery), ophthalmic artery (ethmoidal branches), and ICA (by way of the mandibulo-vidian branch and other arteries arising from the petrous portion, as well as the

Table 1
Fisch classification for JNAs

Classification	Characteristics
Type I	Tumor limited to the nasopharynx and nasal cavity without significant bone destruction
Type II	Tumor invades the pterygopalatine fossa or sinuses with bone destruction
Type IIIa	Tumor invades the infratemporal fossa or orbital region without intracranial involvement
Type IIIb	Tumor invades the infratemporal fossa or orbit without intracranial extradural (parasellar) involvement
Type IVa	Intracranial intradural tumor without infiltration of the cavernous sinus, pituitary fossa, or optic chiasm
Type IVb	Intracranial intradural tumor with infiltration of the cavernous sinus, pituitary fossa, or optic chiasm

Data from Fisch U. The infratemporal fossa approach for nasopharyngeal tumors. Laryngoscope 1983;93(1):36–44; and Roche PH, Paris J, Regis J, et al. Management of invasive juvenile nasopharyngeal angiofibromas: the role of a multimodality approach. Neurosurgery 2007;61(4):768–77 [discussion: 777].

meningohypophyseal trunk and inferolateral trunk). In cases in which the tumor crosses the midline, angiographic examination of the contralateral vascular supply is necessary.[16]

Treatment

Preoperative endovascular embolization followed by surgical removal of the tumor is the treatment modality of choice for extracranial disease.[28,29,30] Radiation therapy is reserved for intracranial extension and unresectable residual or recurrent tumor.[31] Other therapeutic options reported for treatment of JNAs include chemotherapy, cryotherapy, electrocoagulation, injection of sclerosing agents, and treatment using the testosterone-receptor-blocker flutamide.[32]

The surgical approach is predicated on the location of the center of the tumor, the direction of tumor extension, and tumor size.[33,34] Other variables considered in the surgical approach include the effectiveness of the embolization and the surgeon's preference.[28,33] The goal of surgery is to achieve a complete, en bloc, extracapsular resection. Endoscopic resection of small- and medium-sized tumors is technically possible using electocautery, endoscopic visualization, and preoperative embolization.

Preoperative embolization of JNAs is now an accepted means to decrease intraoperative blood loss during surgical resection.[35] Before the use of preoperative embolization, average blood loss for these tumors was noted to be approximately 2000 mL. Moulin and colleagues[36] demonstrated a statistically significant difference in blood loss between embolized and nonembolized surgical groups of patients with high-grade tumors. The benefit of embolization is less clear for smaller, less vascular tumors. Surgical resection of the tumor should be performed from 24 to 72 hours after the embolization to achieve optimal

Table 2
Radkowski surgical staging system for JNAs

Classification	Characteristics
Stage IA	Limited to nose and nasopharyngeal area
Stage IB	Extension into one or more sinuses
Stage IIA	Minimal extension into pterygopalatine fossa
Stage IIB	Occupation of the pterygopalatine fossa without orbital erosion
Stage IIC	Infratemporal fossa extension without cheek or pterygoid plate involvement
Stage IIIA	Erosion of the skull base (middle cranial fossa or pterygoids)
Stage IIIB	Erosion of the skull base with intracranial extension, with or without cavernous sinus involvement

Data from Radkowski D, McGill T, Healy GB, et al. Angiofibroma. Changes in staging and treatment. Arch Otolaryngol Head Neck Surg 1996;122(2):122–9.

devascularization and to prevent recanalization of the occluded arteries or formation of collateral arterial channels.[15,30] The technique of embolization of hypervascular tumors from an endovascular or direct-puncture approach is described in detail in the second section of this article (see Fig. 1).

Complications from transcatheter embolization include cranial nerve palsies due to particulate occlusion of the vasa nervosum of the cranial nerves supplied by the MMA or APAs.[37] Intracranial embolization causing major neurologic complications due to either reflux of embolic particles into the ICA or migration by way of anastomoses between the ECA and ICA has also been reported in a few patients.[38,39,40] One of the most feared complications is central retinal artery occlusion secondary to the presences of dangerous collaterals from the IMA to the intraorbital contents.[41] Migration of a liquid embolic agent into the ophthalmic and middle cerebral artery has also been reported to result from percutaneous direct intratumoral injection of a liquid polymerizing agent in large JNAs.[42]

Radiotherapy is reserved for poor surgical candidates, those who have recurrent or residual disease that is deemed inoperable or large invasive tumors in which surgical removal may threaten vision or require carotid artery resection.[28,31] Potential complications from radiotherapy include brainstem dysfunction, cranial neuropathies, and secondary malignancies of the head and neck.[19] Embolization with radiotherapy has been used with good results for patients who demonstrate residual disease.[28,31]

PARAGANGLIOMAS
Epidemiology

Paragangliomas account for 0.6% of all neoplasms in the head and neck region and 0.03% of all neoplasms.[43] Women are affected four to six times more often than men, and most paragangliomas are diagnosed in individuals between 40 and 60 years of age.[44,45] A higher prevalence of carotid body tumors has been noted in some patients who have chronic obstructive pulmonary disease[46] and in certain populations living at high altitudes (eg, Peruvian Andes, Colorado, and Mexico City); this is believed to be secondary to chronic hypoxia in combination with genetic factors.

Familial paragangliomas have an overall prevalence of 7% to 9%,[47,48] with approximately 90% of cases arising from the carotid body[49] and a higher prevalence occurring in younger patients, with an average age of 38.8 years.[50] The mode of transmission is autosomal dominant, with variable penetrance.[51] Multiple tumors are estimated to occur with an incidence of approximately 10% in nonfamilial cases (see Fig. 3). Multiple lesions occur in familial cases in from 25% to 50% of cases.[52,53]

Clinical Presentation

The clinical symptoms vary according to the size and location of the paraganglioma. Patients may present with a mass lesion in the neck, a cranial nerve deficit, or pulsatile tinnitus.[54] Approximately 1% to 3% of patients will suffer symptoms such as palpitations, hypertension, and flushing caused by vasoactivity from tumor secretion of catecholamines.[55] Patients with a positive family history are at a higher risk for having multicentric disease.

Carotid body paragangliomas (CBPs) usually present as a nontender, insidiously enlarging lateral neck mass in an otherwise asymptomatic patient. The mass can be moved from side to side, can transmit pulsations, and is often associated with a bruit.[56] Other symptoms include hoarseness, stridor, tongue paresis, vertigo, and mild dysphagia.[57]

Jugulotympanic paragangliomas (JTPs) most commonly present with pulsatile tinnitus in association with a retro-tympanic vascular mass (vascular tympanic membrane).[58] Other possible clinical manifestations of these lesions include conductive deafness, vertigo, hoarseness, aural pain, or discharge. Cranial nerve palsies occur late in the course of the disease, resulting in Vernet (jugular foramen) syndrome (motor paralysis of cranial nerves IX, X, and XI),[59] Collect-Sicard syndrome (Vernet syndrome with additional involvement of cranial nerve XII), and Horner syndrome.[60]

Vagal paragangliomas (VPs) manifest as slowly growing, painless lateral neck mass, most commonly located behind the angle of the mandible (83% of cases). Intraoral and neck masses are discovered simultaneously in 46% of cases. Least commonly, VPs may manifest as solitary, intraoral masses with medial displacement of the pretonsillar structures (16% of cases).[43] Vagal nerve deficits are seen late in the clinical course of these lesions.[61] Other lower cranial nerve palsies as a result of hypoglossal, accessory, or glossopharyngeal involvement also commonly occur as late manifestations, typically two years after initial presentation.[62,63] Horner syndrome (ptosis, miosis, anhidrosis, and enophthalmos) with infiltration into the cervical sympathetic chain occurs in 25% of patients.[43] Rare manifestations include isolated hoarseness or vocal cord paralysis.[43]

Behavior and Location

Paragangliomas, also known as glomus tumors or chemodectomas, develop from neural crest cells of the autonomic nervous system. They are highly vascular, benign tumors that are capable of local invasion into the surrounding structures. Only a low percentage (3%) of paragangliomas will transform into malignant tumors.[64]

The site of origin provides the names given to these tumors. They most commonly occur at the carotid bifurcation, in which case they are known as carotid body paragangliomas, or CBPs (see **Figs. 2** and **3**). Additional sites of origin include the jugular bulb (jugular paragangliomas, or JPs); the vagus nerve, usually at the nodose ganglion (vagal paragangliomas, or VPs) (see **Fig. 4**); Jacobsen's nerve within the middle ear mucosa (tympanic paragangliomas, TPs), and other areas, including the aorta and larynx.

CBPs cause splaying of the carotid bifurcation (see **Fig. 2E**). The ICA usually becomes displaced postero-laterally, and the ECA antero-laterally or antero-medially. CBPs can cause encasement of the ICA and ECAs. JTPs can encase the intrapetrous segment of the ICA and extend into the extra- and intradural posterior fossa and even toward the cavernous sinus region. Smaller TPs do not destroy the surrounding bony structures. VPs can extend into the posterior fossa through the jugular foramen. They usually displace the ECA and ICAs antero-medially without splaying the carotid bifurcation.

Histology

The characteristic histologic features of paragangliomas are the zellballen, which are nests of neoplastic chief cells surrounded by reticulin fibers and many blood vessels. Malignancy is not a histologic diagnosis, because both benign and malignant tumors may contain pleomorphic and multinuclear cells and mitoses. Malignancy is a clinical diagnosis, made in cases in which local invasion or metastases are present.[65]

Staging

A comprehensive classification system for CBPs currently widely used in the management of CBPs is shown in **Table 3**.[66]

Classification systems for temporal bone paragangliomas have been proposed by Fisch and Mattox[67] and Jackson.[63] The Fisch classification is shown in **Table 4**. The Glasscock-Jackson classification for JTPs combines the surgical approach with the appearance of the tumor utilizing high-resolution temporal bone CT imaging.

Imaging

Images of paragangliomas produced using CT imaging demonstrate a homogenous and intense enhancement after administration of intravenous contrast material.[45] The typical location of each paraganglioma contributes to the specific diagnosis. CBPs cause splaying of the carotid bifurcation.[45] VPs will cause displacement of the ICA anteriorly.[68] Images of JPs produced using high-resolution CT of the temporal bones usually will show expansion and a moth-eaten-type pattern of erosion of the jugular foramen. Tumor expansion usually occurs superiorly and subsequently into the tympanic cavity, causing destruction of the ossicular chain. Using further enlargement, the tumor may be seen to invade the bony canal of the facial nerve, with possible infiltration of the nerve. Intracranial posterior fossa extension can also occur.[45] TPs are often seen as a small, circumscribed mass at the cochlear promontory.

Table 3
Classification for carotid body tumors with surgical approach and difficulty

Tumor Grade	Carotid Vessel Involvement	Surgical Procedure	Difficulty of Surgical Resection
1	Localized, with minimal adherence to the carotid vessel	Subadventitial approach	Minimal
2	Partial encasement of the carotid vessels	Subadventitial approach	Moderate
3	Surrounds the carotid vessels	Resection, with ICA graft inter position	Surgically challenging, with high risk for operative morbidity

Data from Rao AB, Koeller KK, Adair CF. From the archives of the AFIP. Paragangliomas of the head and neck: radiologic-pathologic correlation. Radiographics 1999;19(6):1605–32; and Hodge KM, Byers RM, Peters LJ. Paragangliomas of the head and neck. Arch Otolaryngol Head Neck Surg 1988;114(8):872–7.

Table 4
Fisch classification of paragangliomas of the temporal bone

Classification	Characteristics
A	Tumors arise along the tympanic plexus on the promontory; confined to the middle ear
B	Tumors arise in the tympanic canal and invade the hypotympanum and mastoid
C	Tumors originate in the dome of the jugular bulb and invade the petrous bone and pyramid; subgroupings C1–4 are based on the degree of erosion of the carotid canal from the carotid foramen to the cavernous sinus
D	Tumors with intracranial extension (posterior fossa); subdivided according to depth of invasion De: extradural 　De1—displacement of the dura <2 cm 　De2—displacement of the dura >2 cm Di: intradural 　Di1—intradural invasion <2 cm 　Di2—intradural invasion >2 cm 　Di3—inoperable

Data from van den Berg R. Imaging and management of head and neck paragangliomas. Eur Radiol 2005;15(7):1310–8; and Fisch U, Mattox D. Paragangliomas of the temporal bone. Microsurgery of the skull base. New York: Thieme Medical; 1988. p. 149–53.

Ossicular destruction is not common; however, it can be seen in larger lesions.[69]

MR imaging is the noninvasive imaging study of choice for paragangliomas because of its excellent soft-tissue contrast compared with CT; however, CT is superior for looking at bone detail. The MR imaging appearance of a paraganglioma is that of a lesion exhibiting low signal intensity on T1-weighted images and a high signal intensity on T2-weighted images. Multiple areas of high and low signal intensity, the so-called "salt and pepper appearance," can be seen within the lesions, as the result of flow-voids from enlarged intratumoral vessels.[70] After the intravenous administration of contrast material, these lesions show rapid and intense homogenous enhancement. The combination of imaging features with the typical localization, typical vessel displacement, enlarged feeding vessels, and intratumoral flow signal makes the diagnosis of a paraganglioma high likely.[54]

Angiographic imaging is usually performed in conjunction with preoperative embolization. The typical angiographic appearance of a paraganglioma is that of a hypervascular mass with enlarged feeding arteries, intense tumor blush, and rapid venous drainage.[71]

CBPs typically splay the ECA and ICA. The APA is the most common feeding vessel identified, although larger lesions may recruit their supply from adjacent ECA branches (eg, the muscular branches of the OA, the ascending cervical artery, the artery of the carotid body, and other unnamed branches of the carotid bifurcation). VPs typically displace the ECA and ICA antero-medially. The vascular supply is similar to that of CBPs; however, bifurcation branches are usually not involved.

Arterial feeders to JPs and TPs include the inferior tympanic branch of the APA, the stylomastoid branch of the OA, the posterior auricular artery, the petrosal branch of the MMA, and the anterior tympanic branch of the IMA.[72] In larger tumors that are invading the skull base, the petrous and cavernous branches of the ICA or the muscular or intracranial branches of the VA may be recruited.[73]

Recently, [111]indium-octreotide, a radioisotope somatostatin analog, has been used to selectively identify paragangliomas. These studies can be used to evaluate for multiple tumors and recurrent or metastatic disease.[74]

Treatment

Treatment options for patients who have paragangliomas include microsurgical resection, radiation therapy, embolization, or any combination of these treatment modalities. The choice of treatment depends on the size, extension, location, and multicentricity of the tumor, along with the patient's age, general health, and symptoms. Complete surgical resection is often possible in young patients with appropriate-sized tumors, and good functional outcome is generally expected. Alternate forms of treatment should be considered for cases in which radical surgical resection carries a high risk for creating a cranial nerve deficit. Radiation therapy is most often used for patients who have tumors with extensive intracranial or skull base involvement, who have multiple or bilateral tumors with potential for postoperative disability from cranial nerve dysfunction, and who have poor surgical risk factors.[53,75] Watchful waiting is another option for an asymptomatic older patient who is not suitable for surgery.

Surgical resection of paragangliomas can be complicated by profuse bleeding caused by the tumors' high vascularity. Preoperative embolization can significantly reduce intraoperative blood loss.[76] This is especially true for VPs and JTPs.[77,78] In patients who have these tumors, a balloon occlusion test is also often requested by the operating surgeon to evaluate the adequacy of the intracranial collateral network and to assess if the patient may be able to tolerate the sacrifice of the ICA during radical surgery. The benefit of performing preoperative embolization for patients who have small CBPs and TPs is questionable; however, a statistically significant difference in operative blood loss has been shown for patients who had CBPs with diameters larger than 3.0 cm and who underwent preoperative embolization.[71] The technique of embolization of hypervascular tumors from an endovascular or direct-puncture approach is described in detail in the second section (paragraph eight) of this article. In the case of single-compartment tumors, the entire lesion may be embolized through one feeding vessel. Multicompartmental tumors require selective catheterization and embolization of each individual feeder.

As with other hypervascular head and neck tumors, stroke is a potential complication from embolization using an endovascular or direct-puncture approach. In paragangliomas, the posterior circulation is at greatest risk because of the rich collaterals between the VA and the C1, C2, and C3 branches of the OA and the APA. Other complications related to these lesions that can result from transcatheter embolization include cranial nerve palsies as the result of particulate occlusion of the vasa nervosum of the cranial nerves supplied by the MMA, OA, and APAs. The facial nerve is at highest risk.[79]

UNIVERSITY OF MICHIGAN EXPERIENCE

Over the last six years (2002–2008), 85 patients who had hypervascular head and neck tumors underwent preoperative embolization at the University of Michigan by the two coauthors (Gandhi and Gemmete). A total of 89 procedures were performed in these 85 patients because two patients with large JNAs needed to have two procedures each and another patient with an extensive endolymphatic sac tumor had to be embolized in three stages to facilitate a staged resection. All of the patients who had embolized tumors underwent subsequent surgical resection, and the estimated blood loss for each resection ranged from 50 to 2400 cc. The most commonly embolized tumors in the series were paragangliomas (n = 39), and the mean blood loss for these tumors was 510 cc.

There was one major complication, which was in a patient after preoperative embolization of a large, 6-cm CBP. The patient suffered contralateral visual loss and small emboli in the brain. This patient had a previously undiagnosed large patent foramen ovale (PFO). Given that the incidence of PFOs in autopsy studies is reported to be fairly high (12%–35%) and that the clinical reports of patients younger than 55 years of age state that unexplained stroke due to PFO occurs in 12% to 41% of the population studied,[80] preoperative screening of patients using a bubble-contrast echocardiogram may be helpful in avoiding this complication. Additionally, if a large shunt is discovered in the tumor, the arteriovenous shunt can be occluded using coils and the particles can be upsized to from 500 to 700 μm to prevent passage into the venous system.

At the University of Michigan Health System, two of the coauthors routinely employ neurophysiologic monitoring under general anesthesia in the patients with larger, complex, hypervascular masses as well as those with significant skull base involvement. The information provided by brainstem auditory evoked potentials, somatosensory evoked potentials, and electroencephalographic results can help alert the physician to unexpected embolic events or changes in cerebral perfusion.

Over the last two years, the two coauthors have also increasingly been using direct percutaneous injection of either n-BCA or Onyx into the tumor bed. They believe a more complete devascularization of the tumor can be achieved by injecting liquid embolic agents from a percutaneous injection into the tumor. Direct intratumoral injection allows easy access to the tumor bed and overcomes limitations that can result from arterial tortuosity, the small size of the arterial feeders, atherosclerotic disease, or catheter-induced vasospasm.

SUMMARY

A detailed understanding of the functional anatomy of the ECA is essential for safe and effective endovascular therapy for hypervascular tumors of the head and neck. The recent development of newer particulate materials and percutaneous techniques using new liquid embolic agents may allow for a more complete devascularization of tumors. Nontarget embolization of the central retinal artery and anterior intracranial circulation is of concern when performing transcatheter embolization of JNAs. In patients who have paragangliomas, the posterior intracranial circulation and cranial nerves are at greatest risk for nontarget embolization. However, the incidence of the complications is extremely low for surgeons who have meticulous technique and detailed understanding of head and neck vascular anatomy and potential collateral pathways.

REFERENCES

1. Smith TP. Embolization in the external carotid artery. J Vasc Interv Radiol 2006;17(12):1897–912.
2. Jenson ME. Endovascular and percutaneous therapy for extracranial tumors. In: Marks MP, Do HM, editors. Endovascular and percutaneous therapy of the brain and spine. Philadelphia: Lippincott Williams & Wilkins; 2002. p. 361–88.
3. Russell EJ. Functional angiography of the head and neck. AJNR Am J Neuroradiol 1986;7(5):927–36.
4. Horton JA, Kerber CW. Lidocaine injection into external carotid branches: provocative test to preserve cranial nerve function in therapeutic embolization. AJNR Am J Neuroradiol 1986;7(1):105–8.
5. Deveikis JP. Sequential injections of amobarbital sodium and lidocaine for provocative neurologic testing in the external carotid circulation. AJNR Am J Neuroradiol 1996;17(6):1143–7.
6. Valavanis A, Christoforidis G. Applications of interventional neuroradiology in the head and neck. Semin Roentgenol 2000;35(1):72–83.
7. Kai Y, Hamada J, Morioka M, et al. Appropriate interval between embolization and surgery in patients with meningioma. AJNR Am J Neuroradiol 2002;23(1):139–42.
8. Chun JY, McDermott MW, Lamborn KR, et al. Delayed surgical resection reduces intraoperative blood loss for embolized meningiomas. Neurosurgery 2002;50(6):1231–5 [discussion: 1235–7].
9. Dean BL, Flom RA, Wallace RC, et al. Efficacy of endovascular treatment of meningiomas: evaluation with matched samples. AJNR Am J Neuroradiol 1994;15(9):1675–80.
10. Wakhloo AK, Juengling FD, Delthoven VV. Extended preoperative polyvinyl alcohol microembolization of intracranial meningiomas: assessment of two embolization techniques. AJNR Am J Neuroradiol 1993;14(3):571–82.
11. Kallmes DF, Evans AJ, Kaptain GJ, et al. Hemorrhagic complications in embolization of a meningioma: case report and review of the literature. Neuroradiology 1997;39(12):877–80.
12. Quadros RS, Gallas S, Delcourt C, et al. Preoperative embolization of a cervicodorsal paraganglioma by direct percutaneous injection of onyx and endovascular delivery of particles. AJNR Am J Neuroradiol 2006;27(9):1907–9.
13. Abud DG, Mounayer C, Benndorf G, et al. Intratumoral injection of cyanoacrylate glue in head and neck paragangliomas. AJNR Am J Neuroradiol 2004;25(9):1457–62.
14. Mehra YN, Mann SB, Dubey SP, et al. Computed tomography for determining pathways of extension and a staging and treatment system for juvenile angiofibromas. Ear Nose Throat J 1989;68(8):576–89.
15. Davis KR. Embolization of epistaxis and juvenile nasopharyngeal angiofibromas. AJR Am J Roentgenol 1987;148(1):209–18.
16. Berenstein A, Lasjaunias P, ter Brugge KG. editors. Surgical neuroangiography. 2nd edition. Clinical and endovascular treatment aspects in adults. vol. 2.1. New York: Springer-Verlag; 2004. p. 201–26.
17. Apostol JV, Frazell EL. Juvenile nasopharyngeal angiofibroma: a clinical study. Cancer 1965;18: 869–78.
18. Buetow PC, Smirniotopoulos JG, Wenig BM. Pediatric sinonasal tumors. Appl Radiol 1993;22:21–8.
19. Gantz B, Seid AB, Weber RS. Nasopharyngeal angiofibroma. Head Neck 1992;14(1):67–71.
20. Batsakis J, Klopp C, Newman W. Fibrosarcoma arising in a juvenile nasopharyngeal angiofibroma following extensive radiation therapy. Am Surg 1955;21(8):786–93.
21. Gisselsson L, Lindgren M, Stenram U. Sarcomatous transformation of a juvenile nasopharyngeal angiofibroma. Acta Pathol Microbiol Scand 1958;42(4): 305–12.
22. Weprin LS, Seimers PT. Spontaneous regression of juvenile nasopharyngeal angiofibroma. Arch Otolaryngol Head Neck Surg 1991;117(7):796–9.
23. Thompson LDR, Fanburg-Smith JC. Tumours of the nasopharynx: nasopharyngeal angiofibroma. In: Barnes L, Eveson JW, Reichart P, et al, editors. World Health Organization Classification of Tumours. Pathology & genetics head and neck tumours. Lyon (France): IARC Press; 2005. p. 102–3.
24. Fisch U. The infratemporal fossa approach for nasopharyngeal tumors. Laryngoscope 1983;93(1):36–44.
25. Radkowski D, McGill T, Healy GB, et al. Angiofibroma. Changes in staging and treatment. Arch Otolaryngol Head Neck Surg 1996;122(2):122–9.
26. Sessions RB, Bryan RN, Naclerio RM, et al. Radiographic staging of juvenile angiofibroma. Head Neck Surg 1981;3(4):279–83.
27. Ungkanont K, Byers RM, Weber RS, et al. Juvenile nasopharyngeal angiofibroma: an update of therapeutic management. Head Neck 1996;18(1):60–6.

28. Roche PH, Paris J, Regis J, et al. Management of invasive juvenile nasopharyngeal angiofibromas: the role of a multimodality approach. Neurosurgery 2007;61(4):768–77 [discussion: 777].

29. Deschler DG, Kaplan MJ, Boles R. Treatment of large juvenile nasopharyngeal angiofibroma. Otolaryngol Head Neck Surg 1992;106(3):278–84.

30. Gullane PJ, Davidson J, O'Dwyer T, et al. Juvenile angiofibroma: a review of the literature and a case series report. Laryngoscope 1992;102(8):928–33.

31. Fields JN, Halverson KJ, Devineni VR, et al. Juvenile nasopharyngeal angiofibroma: efficacy of radiation therapy. Radiology 1990;176:263–5.

32. Gates GA, Rice DH, Koopman CF, et al. Flutamide-induced regression of angiofibroma. Laryngoscope 1992;102(6):641–4.

33. Fagan JJ, Snyderman CH, Carrau RL, et al. Nasopharyngeal angiofibromas: selecting a surgical approach. Head Neck 1997;19(5):391–9.

34. Jorissen M, Eloy P, Rombaux P, et al. Endoscopic sinus surgery for juvenile nasopharyngeal angiofibromas. Acta Otorhinolaryngol Belg 2000;54(2):201–19.

35. Garcia-Cervigon E, Bien S, Rufenacht D, et al. Preoperative embolization of naso-pharyngeal angiofibromas. Report of 58 cases. Neuroradiology 1988;30(6):556–60.

36. Moulin G, Chagnaud C, Gras R, et al. Juvenile nasopharyngeal angiofibroma: comparison of blood loss during removal in embolized group versus nonembolized group. Cardiovasc Intervent Radiol 1995;18(3):158–61.

37. Gupta AK, Purkayastha S, Bodhey NK, et al. Preoperative embolization of hypervascular head and neck tumours. Australas Radiol 2007;51(5):446–52.

38. TerBrugge KG, Lasjaunias P, Chiu MC. Super-selective angiography and embolization of skull base tumors. Can J Neurol Sci 1985;12(4):341–4.

39. Valvanis A. Preoperative embolization of the head and neck: indications, patient selection, goals, and precautions. AJNR Am J Neuroradiol 1986;7(5):943–52.

40. Mehta BA, Jack CR Jr, Boulos RS, et al. Interventional neuroradiology: Henry Ford Hospital experience with transcatheter embolization of vascular lesions in the head, neck, and spine. Henry Ford Hosp Med J 1986;34(1):19–30.

41. Mames RN, Snady-McCoy L, Guy J. Central retinal and posterior ciliary artery occlusion after particle embolization of the external carotid artery system. Ophthalmology 1991;98(4):527–31.

42. Casasco A, Houdart E, Biondi A, et al. Major complications of percutaneous embolization of skull-base tumors. AJNR Am J Neuroradiol 1999;20(1):179–81.

43. Borba LA, Al-Mefty O. Intravagal paragangliomas: report of four cases. Neurosurgery 1996;38(3):569–75.

44. Tasar M, Yetiser S. Glomus tumors: therapeutic role of selective embolization. J Craniofac Surg 2004;15(3):497–505.

45. Rao AB, Koeller KK, Adair CF. From the archives of the AFIP. Paragangliomas of the head and neck: radiologic-pathologic correlation. Radiographics 1999;19(6):1605–32.

46. Saldana MJ, Salem LE, Travezan R. High altitude hypoxia and chemodectomas. Hum Pathol 1973;4(2):251–63.

47. Parry DM, Li FP, Strong LC, et al. Carotid body tumors in humans: genetics and epidemiology. J Natl Cancer Inst 1982;68(4):573–8.

48. Zaslav AL, Myssiorek D, Mucia C, et al. Cytogenetic analysis of tissues from patients with familial paragangliomas of the head and neck. Head Neck 1995;17(2):102–7.

49. Lawson W. Glomus bodies and tumors. N Y State J Med 1980;80(10):1567–75.

50. Grufferman S, Gillman MW, Pasternak LP, et al. Familial carotid body tumors: case report and epidemiologic review. Cancer 1980;46(9):2116–22.

51. van Baars F, Cremers C, van den Broek P, et al. Genetic aspects of nonchromaffin paraganglioma. Hum Genet 1982;60(4):305–9.

52. Gulya AJ. The glomus tumor and its biology. Laryngoscope 1993;103(11 Pt 2 Suppl 60):7–15.

53. Jackson CG. Neurotologic skull base surgery for glomus tumors. Diagnosis for treatment planning and treatment options. Laryngoscope 1993;103(11 Pt 2 Suppl 60):17–22.

54. van den Berg R. Imaging and management of head and neck paragangliomas. Eur Radiol 2005;15(7):1310–8.

55. Kliewer KE, Cochran AJ. A review of the histology, ultrastructure, immunohistology, and molecular biology of extra-adrenal paragangliomas. Arch Pathol Lab Med 1989;113(11):1209–18 [erratum in: Arch Pathol Lab Med 1990;114(3):308].

56. ReMine WH, Weiland LH, ReMine SG. Carotid body tumors: chemodectomas. Curr Probl Cancer 1978;2(12):1–27.

57. Bishop GB Jr, Urist MM, el Gammal T, et al. Paragangliomas of the neck. Arch Surg 1992;127(12):1441–5.

58. Remley KB, Coit WE, Harnsberger HR, et al. Pulsatile tinnitus and the vascular tympanic membrane: CT, MR, and angiographic findings. Radiology 1990;174(2):383–9.

59. Spector GJ, Druck NS, Gado M. Neurologic manifestations of glomus tumors in the head and neck. Arch Neurol 1976;33(4):270–4.

60. Makek M, Franklin DJ, Zhao JC, et al. Neural infiltration of glomus temporale tumors. Am J Otol 1990;11(1):1–5.

61. Murphy TE, Huvos AG, Frazell EL. Chemodectomas of the glomus intravagale: vagal body tumors, nonchromaffin paragangliomas of the nodose ganglion of the vagus nerve. Ann Surg 1970;172(2):246–55.

62. Arts HA, Fagan PA. Vagal body tumors. Otolaryngol Head Neck Surg 1991;105(1):78–85.

63. Jackson CG. Basic surgical principles of neurotologic skull base surgery. Laryngoscope 1993; 103(11 Pt 2 Suppl 60):29–44.

64. Manolidis S, Shohet JA, Jackson CG, et al. Malignant glomus tumors. Laryngoscope 1999;109(1):30–4.

65. Barnes L, Eveson JW, Reichart PA, et al, editors. World Health Organization classification of tumours: pathology and genetics of head and neck tumours. Lyon (France): IARC Press; 2005. p. 361–70.

66. Hodge KM, Byers RM, Peters LJ. Paragangliomas of the head and neck. Arch Otolaryngol Head Neck Surg 1988;114(8):872–7.

67. Fisch U, Mattox D. Paragangliomas of the temporal bone. Microsurgery of the skull base. New York: Thieme Medical; 1988. p. 149–53.

68. Som PM, Biller HF, Lawson W, et al. Parapharyngeal space masses: an updated protocol based upon 104 cases. Radiology 1984;153(1):149–56.

69. Noujain SE, Pattekar MA, Cacciarelli A, et al. Paraganglioma of the temporal bone: role of magnetic resonance imaging versus computed tomography. Top Magn Reson Imaging 2000;11(2):108–22.

70. Olsen WL, Dillion WP, Kelly WM, et al. MR imaging of paragangliomas. AJR Am J Roentgenol 1987; 148(1):201–4.

71. Tikkakoski T, Loutonen J, Leinonen S, et al. Preoperative embolization in the management of neck paragangliomas. Laryngoscope 1997;107(6):821–6.

72. Moret J, Delvert G, Bretonneau CH, et al. Vascularization of the ear: normal-variations-glomus tumors. J Neuroradiol 1982;9(3):209–60.

73. Jordan CE, Newton TH. Internal carotid artery supply to temporal bone chemodectomas. Neuroradiology 1975;8(5):253–7.

74. Kwekkeboom DJ, van Urk H, Pauw BK, et al. Octreotide scintigraphy for the detection of paragangliomas. J Nucl Med 1993;34(6):873–8.

75. Carrasco V, Rosenman J. Radiation therapy of glomus jugulare tumors. Laryngoscope 1993; 103(11 Pt 2 Suppl 60):23–7.

76. Robison JG, Shagets FW, Beckett WC, et al. A multidisciplinary approach to reducing morbidity and operative blood loss during resection of carotid body tumor. Surg Gynecol Obstet 1989;168(2):166–70.

77. Murphy TP, Brackmann DE. Effects of preoperative embolization on glomus jugulare tumors. Laryngoscope 1989;99(12):1244–7.

78. Persky MS, Setton A, Niimi Y, et al. Combined endovascular and surgical treatment of head and neck paragangliomas—a team approach. Head Neck 2002;24(5):423–31.

79. Marangos N, Schumacher M. Facial palsy after glomus jugulare tumor embolization. J Laryngol Otol 1999;113(2):268–70.

80. Kerut EK, Norfleet WT, Plotnick GD, et al. Patent foramen ovale: a review of associated conditions and the impact of physiological size. J Am Coll Cardiol 2001;38:613–23.

Neurointerventional Management of Low-Flow Vascular Malformations of the Head and Neck

David J. Choi, MD, PhD[a], Ahmad I. Alomari, MD[b],
Gulraiz Chaudry, MD[b], Darren B. Orbach, MD, PhD[c,*]

KEYWORDS

- Low-flow vascular malformation • Venous malformation
- Lymphatic malformation • Capillary malformation
- Sclerotherapy • Syndromic vascular anomalies

Mulliken and Glowacki's[1] seminal classification of vascular anomalies into vascular tumors (with infantile hemangiomas being paradigmatic) versus nontumorous vascular malformations has been as important in the head and neck region as elsewhere. These latter are congenital, have an equal gender incidence, virtually always grow in size with the patient during childhood, and virtually never involute spontaneously. The vascular malformations can in turn be subclassified into high-flow (ie, those with arterial components, such as arteriovenous malformations and fistulae) and low-flow (ie, those with no arterial components). Our focus here is entirely on the latter, the low-flow malformations, which include those with venous, lymphatic, and, to a lesser extent, capillary components. We address diagnostic and clinical characteristics, particularly insofar as they relate to the structures of the head and neck, and discuss neurointerventional management in some detail.

CLINICOPATHOLOGIC FEATURES
Capillary Malformations

Capillary malformations or stains, of which the facial port wine stain is the best known example, are flat, well demarcated, lesions, pink in infancy and tending to darken to purple with age (Fig. 1A). These are to be differentiated from the very common fading macular stains (the "stork bite" and "angel kiss" being the most well known), which typically lighten or disappear. Histopathology demonstrates ectatic blood vessels in the dermis associated with reduction in innervation, which may play a role in the pathogenesis.[2] Overall, there is a reported incidence of 0.3% at birth, with no known gender or ethnic predilections.[3,4] They may be single or multiple, and have a predilection for the head and neck region.

Capillary stains may occur in a dermatomal configuration, most commonly corresponding to the V1 and V2 branches of the trigeminal nerve (Fig. 1B). Whereas in most cases, the trigeminal dermatomal distribution occurs in isolation, in 3% to 8% of patients, there is an association with Sturge Weber syndrome and unilateral glaucoma.[5,6] In the vast majority of cases with neuroocular involvement, the capillary malformation occurs in the V1 distribution, with or without involvement of V2 and V3.[5,6]

[a] Division of Neuroradiology, Brigham and Women's Hospital, Harvard Medical School, 75 Francis Street, PBB 356, Boston, MA 02115, USA
[b] Division of Interventional Radiology, Children's Hospital Boston, Harvard Medical School, 300 Longwood Avenue, Boston, MA 02115, USA
[c] Division of Neurointerventional Radiology, Children's Hospital Boston, Brigham and Women's Hospital, Harvard Medical School, 75 Francis Street, PBB 356, Boston, MA 02115, USA
* Corresponding author.
E-mail address: dorbach@partners.org (D.B. Orbach).

Neuroimag Clin N Am 19 (2009) 199–218
doi:10.1016/j.nic.2009.01.003
1052-5149/09/$ – see front matter © 2009 Elsevier Inc. All rights reserved.

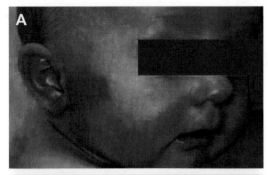

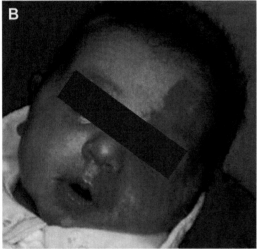

Fig. 1. Capillary stains. (A) Flat, pink lesion just anterior to the right ear. (B) Capillary cutaneous stains in the distribution of the V1 and V2 branches of the left trigeminal nerve.

Several syndromes include capillary stains within their list of clinical manifestations, the most familiar being Sturge-Weber syndrome; other examples (not necessarily involving head and neck capillary stains) are Klippel-Trenaunay syndrome, Parkes Weber syndrome, macrocephaly-capillary malformation syndrome, and capillary malformation-arteriovenous malformation syndrome (CM-AVM). CM-AVM has been recently linked to chromosome 5q14-21, with a defect in the RASA1 gene,[7] which encodes a p120 Ras GTPase-activating protein, involved in cell adhesion and angiogenesis.[8] Capillary malformations can be associated with overgrowth of the affected limb and even with hemihypertrophy. Klippel-Trenaunay syndrome consists of limb overgrowth with capillary malformation, venous anomalies, such as phlebectasia and hypoplasia, and lymphatic malformations.

In the vast majority of cases, capillary stains are only of clinical import because of issues of cosmesis and because of their syndromic association, although they have been reported to very rarely

bleed profusely after minor trauma. Given the superficial nature of the lesions, imaging is typically done to exclude associated deeper lesions and associated neuro-ocular abnormalities, rather than to assess the capillary stain itself. Doppler ultrasound may be useful in cases where a deeper arteriovenous malformation is suspected. The current standard treatment is pulsed-dye laser, although only 15% to 20% of lesions clear completely. This technique has been reviewed elsewhere.[9]

Venous Malformations

Venous malformations (VM) are congenital anomalies characterized by irregular endothelial-lined channels, with thin walls deficient in smooth muscle.[1] When superficial enough to be appreciated externally, they typically have a bluish purplish hue, and are soft and compressible (Fig. 2A, B). Head and neck venous malformations often expand when the patient is head-down, during Valsalva, and during other maneuvers that reduce venous return. Episodic focal thrombosis is nearly ubiquitous and may be associated with swelling and pain. Permanent phleboliths resulting from such episodes are common. The overall incidence of venous malformations is approximately 1 per 10,000.[10] They are equally likely to occur in the head and neck region and in the extremities, with 40% found in each, with the remaining 20% seen in the trunk.[11] As with other vascular malformations, swelling and enlargement can occur following trauma or hormonal changes, such as menarche or pregnancy.

Pain associated with venous malformations is complex and multifactorial. Other than the above-mentioned thrombosis, intra-articular hemorrhage, muscle fibrosis, and bone and muscle deformity resulting in premature arthropathy can all serve as etiologies for pain and discomfort. In the head and neck in particular, the extent of the lesion is often greater than appreciated on clinical examination. Facial venous malformations frequently demonstrate extension into the deeper musculature and oral mucosa, and can present with oral bleeding (Fig. 2C–E). Similarly, there is often extension of temporal venous malformations into the parotid gland, and of neck venous malformations into the larynx or trepezius.[4] Additional clinical manifestations typically relate to mass effect from a growing lesion within or adjacent to an important anatomic space, such as the orbit or airway (Fig. 3A, Fig. 2B). Cosmesis is often an issue as well, with facial asymmetry inducing patients or their parents to seek treatment.

Venous malformations are associated with several syndromes, including glomuvenous

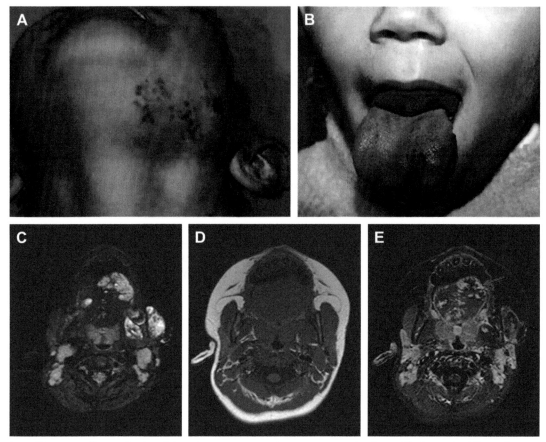

Fig. 2. Venous malformation involving the tongue, masticator space, and submandibular and sublingual spaces. (*A, B*) Purplish compressible lesion that enlarges with Valsalva or dependent positioning. Axial STIR (*C*) and pre- (*D*) and post-contrast T1-weighted images (the latter with fat suppression) (*E*), illustrating T2 hyperintensity throughout the lesion, with variable enhancement (*single anterior arrow* at the tongue versus *two lateral posterior arrows* at the masseter and pterygoid).

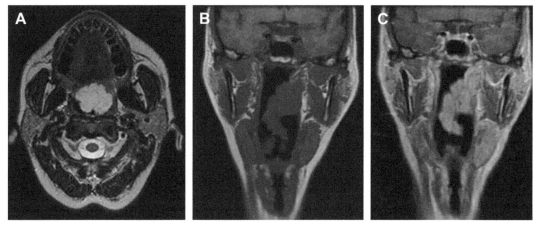

Fig. 3. Venous malformation that involved the soft palate, nasopharynx, and oropharynx. Note the significant airway narrowing. The patient presented with intermittent sleep apnea and occasional dysphagia. Axial post-contrast T1-weighted image (*A*) and coronal pre- (*B*) and post-contrast (*C*) T1-weighted images demonstrate avid and homogeneous enhancement of the venous malformation in this case.

malformation (glomulin mutation), cutaneomucosal venous malformation (TIE2 mutation), and blue rubber bleb nevus syndrome.[12,13] Blue rubber bleb is a sporadic disorder with a plethora of venous malformations in the head and neck (Fig. 4) as well as in the extremities (Fig. 5), with the development of new lesions throughout life.

As manifestations of dysplastic veins, venous malformations by definition drain into the regional normal venous system. Given the typically large caliber of the anomalous venous sac relative to its low inflow, as well as the typically diminutive connectors between the malformation and adjacent normal veins, venous drainage is often delayed; rapid drainage can, however, occur. As we shall see, the rapidity, type, and particular pathway of venous drainage impacts on management strategy.

Lymphatic Malformations

Lymphatic malformations (LM) consist of cysts that are classified as either macrocystic, microcystic, or combined. Although strict numerical criteria for macrocysts have been proposed, we prefer to define as macrocystic any radiologically discernible cyst. As will be described later in this article, both the imaging characteristics and the response to treatment hinge crucially upon this distinction. Lymphatic malformations are particularly transspatial, crossing tissue planes and regional boundaries. The overlying skin or mucosal surfaces may demonstrate lymphatic vesicles (in microcystic cases).

Macrocystic lymphatic malformations have a decided predilection for the head and neck region, manifesting there 70% to 80% of the time; other locations include axillae in 20%, superior mediastinum, mesentery, retroperitoneum,

pelvis, and lower limbs. Although they are congenital lesions, lymphatic malformations may not present immediately after birth (Fig. 6). Clinical manifestations typically appear before the second year of life, however, owing to increasing mass effect. Sudden enlargement may follow infection or intralesional hemorrhage. Spontaneous involution, although unusual, has been reported.[14] Numerous syndromes have been reported in association with LM, including Klippel-Trenaunay, Turner, Noonan, and trisomies 13 and 18.[11] The incidence of lymphatic malformations is approximately 2.8 per 100,000 hospital admissions,[15] but there are no accepted figures for overall population incidence.

Morbidity associated with lymphatic malformations in the head and neck is primarily through recurrent infection, tissue overgrowth, mass effect on functionally important structures, skeletal hypertrophy,[16] and via effects on cosmesis. In rare cases outside the head and neck, morbidity can be related to fluid depletion from massive chylous collections in the thorax or abdomen, or to functional impairment from diffuse lower extremity involvement.

Combined and Syndromic Low-Flow Malformations

Although frequently diagnosed in clinical imaging reports, the true incidence of combined or syndromic vascular anomalies, while unknown, is almost certainly very low. The frequent misdiagnosis results from atypical clinical and imaging appearance of a lesion (eg, a microcystic LM mimicking a VM, although not manifesting the classic imaging findings). Klippel-Trenaunay patients have all three major types of malformation

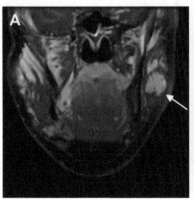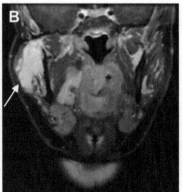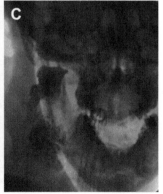

Fig. 4. Blue rubber bleb nevus syndrome, with bilateral masseteric venous malformations. The patient had additional lesions on one forearm and the contralateral leg. The masseteric malformations were intermittently symptomatic, primarily causing pain, which responded well to sclerotherapy. (A, B) Coronal post-contrast T1-weighted MR with fat suppression. Only the symptomatic lesion was treated (C).

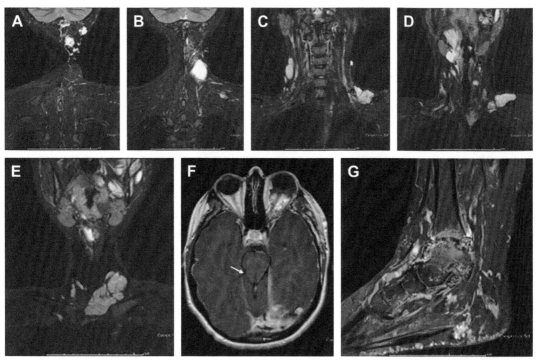

Fig. 5. Blue rubber bleb nevus syndrome. (*A–E*) Successive coronal STIR images demonstrate a complex venous malformation extending from the occiput posteriorly to the thoracic inlet at the suprasternal notch anteriorly, and involving the neck bilaterally. (*F*) Post-contrast axial T1-weighted image demonstrates intraconal, post-septal venous malformation in the left orbit; the patient's vision and extraocular movements remained intact. Incidentally noted is tectal beaking; the patient additionally has positional headaches and cerebellar tonsillar ectopia. (*G*) Diffuse venous malformation involving the ankle in the same patient.

present in the affected limb; hence the name capillary-lymphatic-venous malformations (CLVM).

DIAGNOSIS: IMAGING CHARACTERISTICS

Low-flow vascular malformations can often be correctly diagnosed based on physical examination and history. Anomalous draining veins of venous malformations can on occasion be seen superficially, and VMs tend to be compressible, have a characteristic bluish color, and to expand when venous drainage is slowed. Lymphatic malformations are soft, noncompressible translucent masses with overlying normal or bluish skin, often with superficial vesicles (in microcystic cases). Nevertheless, imaging plays an essential role in characterizing these lesions to confirm the diagnosis (such as excluding the diagnosis of neoplasm), to define the spatial extent of the lesion and its relationship to important nearby structures, and for treatment planning.[10,11]

Superficial and small lesions are well examined by ultrasound, with gray scale studies defining the extent and compressibility of the lesion, and spectral and color Doppler interrogation used to identify the flow characteristics.[11] Sonography can also play a crucial role in differentiating macrocystic and microcystic lymphatic malformation (Fig. 6D). Very superficial lesions may be remarkably inconspicuous on MR imaging and yet well defined on ultrasound. Additionally, ultrasound has significant utility in providing image guidance for sclerotherapy, as described below.

However, in most cases, we have found MR imaging to be virtually indispensible. Its unparalleled contrast resolution more reliably determines the full extent of the lesion than any other modality. We most heavily rely on pre- and post-contrast T1-weighted images as well as T2-weighted images, and consider fat suppression to be critical in all MR sequences in the workup of vascular anomalies (see Fig. 6). Other MR techniques, such as MR angiography, venography, and lymphangiography, tend to contribute little in cases of low-flow anomalies. CT plays more of an adjunctive role in the workup of vascular malformations, being of most use in cases where bony involvement is crucial to delineate (as in sinus, skull base, cranium, or mandibular cases).

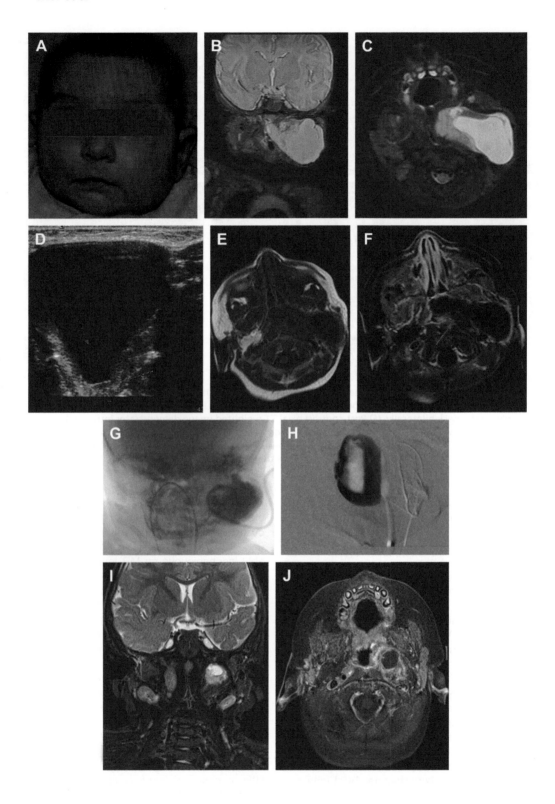

Untreated, both venous and lymphatic malformations typically appear hyperintense on T2 imaging, and the scope of the abnormal T2 signal can be used to define the overall extent of the lesion. After treatment by sclerotherapy, with the resultant progressive conversion of lesion to scar tissue, the T2 signal characteristically becomes less hyperintense. The enhancement pattern after contrast administration is a crucial differentiating feature, with venous malformations most characteristically enhancing avidly but in a patchy, heterogeneous pattern (see **Figs. 2** to **4**). In contrast, enhancement of lymphatic malformations is variable (see **Fig. 6**). Mild rim enhancement may be seen with macrocystic lymphatic malformations, with only minimal enhancement identified in microcystic LMs (**Fig. 7**); however, in the setting of superinfection or inflammation, LMs may enhance avidly as well.

Venous malformations often display irregular intervening venous walls within the hyperintense areas, and occasionally adjacent enhancing serpentine vascular channels can be seen.[17] Thrombi can have variable appearances, based on their age. Phleboliths are hypointense on all sequences on MR, are dense on CT, and are typically mobile (although confined to the venous space). They are hyperechoic and show acoustic shadowing on ultrasound. Although phleboliths have been thought to be virtually pathognomonic of venous malformations, they can rarely occur in lymphatic malformations as well.[18] Venous malformations typically show compressible, confluent anechoic-hypoechoic channels on ultrasound (which are demonstrably venous on color Doppler imaging), separated by more solid regions of variable echogenicity (**Fig. 8**).

The sonographic appearance of lymphatic malformations is dependent upon the type. Macrocystic lymphatic malformations show anechoic cysts, often containing internal debris or fluid-fluid levels resulting from episodes of hemorrhage. Internal septations are common and best visualized with sonography (**Fig. 9**). Microcystic lymphatic malformations are ill-defined echoge-nic masses, showing diffuse involvement of surrounding tissue. On MR, macrocysts are T2 hyperintense and T1 hypointense, whereas on CT they are hypodense. On both MR and CT, the imaging characteristics may be altered by intracystic hemorrhage. There is variable enhancement of cyst septations on both MR and CT (see **Fig. 9**). In both modalities, microcystic LMs often have some degree of heterogeneous enhancement and ill-defined borders.

IMAGE-GUIDED TREATMENT
General Comments

Head and neck vascular malformations are relatively rare, and patients benefit from treatment by multidisciplinary teams, ideally at centers coordinated for treatment of these complex lesions.[19] Specialists involved in the care of head and neck vascular malformations include plastic surgeons, interventional and neurointerventional radiologists, otolaryngologists, ophthalmologists, neurosurgeons, hematologists, pediatricians, dermatologists, and social workers.

At our institution, the primary mode of treatment for low-flow vascular malformations is via percutaneous sclerotherapy. This involves the injection, under imaging guidance, of an agent that induces endothelial damage, typically elicits an avid inflammatory response (**Fig. 10**S), and finally leads to thrombosis (in venous malformations) and fibrosis. These latter effects may not be seen for several weeks. In our practice, surgery is reserved for resection of residual portions that continue to present some degree of functional impairment owing to mass effect, for lesions recalcitrant to interventional techniques, and for cosmesis, to improve contour symmetry. In rare instances, surgery is used as a first step in treatment, to compartmentalize large lesions as an aid to

Fig. 6. Lymphatic malformation involving the left parotid, parapharyngeal, and submandibular spaces. (A) Only a subtle contour asymmetry is present clinically, with slight prominence of the left cheek relative to the right. Coronal (B) and axial (C) T2-weighted images show the large macrocystic component as homogeneously hyperintense. Note the narrowed airway. (D) Sonography demonstrates the large echolucent macrocyst. Dot-dash arrow illustrates a sediment-fluid level, consistent with prior hemorrhage or proteinaceous debris. Dashed arrow illustrates the echogenic, deeper component, likely microcystic. (E, F) Pre-contrast and post-contrast, fat-suppressed T1-weighed axial images demonstrate enhancement of the deep medial component of the LM, with characteristic ill-defined borders (red arrow). (G) Left anterior oblique fluoroscopic image demonstrating a pig-tail catheter within the macrocystic component. (H) Subtraction image using road-mapping technique displays injection into the macrocyst in real-time. (I, J) Follow-up MR imaging demonstrates near complete regression of the macrocystic component. Remnant is the microcystic, most medial component of the LM, showing characteristics of solid tissue on both coronal T2 (I) and axial post-contrast, fat-suppressed (J) images. Airway impingement is markedly improved.

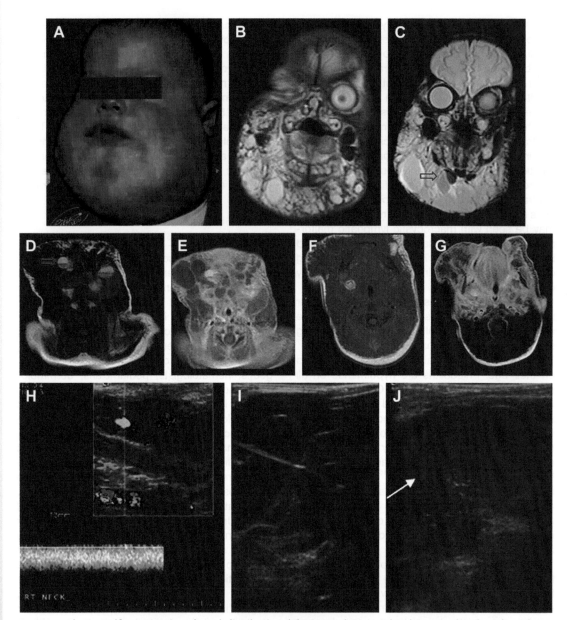

Fig. 7. Lymphatic malformation in a beard distribution (A). Coronal T2-weighted images (B, C) and axial pre-contrast (D, F) and post-contrast (E, G) T1-weighted images demonstrate a large lymphatic malformation with numerous macrocysts and a substantial microcystic component. Some macrocysts demonstrate fluid-fluid levels (open arrows in C and D). Solid arrow in G demonstrates the irregularly defined enhancing component characteristic of microcystic LM. (H) Color Doppler sonography demonstrates vessels traversing the septae and surrounding the cystic regions, as is frequently seen in LM. (I, J) Sonography during sclerotherapy demonstrates the needle within a macrocyst. Injected sclerosant has a characteristic mobile echogenic appearance (arrow in J). Two sessions of sclerotherapy (K, L) and (M, N) demonstrate successive opacification of the macrocysts.

sclerotherapy (Fig. 8I) or to place a tracheostomy for airway lesions.[20]

For percutaneous sclerotherapy, the lesion is cannulated using an angiocatheter or a needle under ultrasound or fluoroscopic guidance.[21] MR guidance for needle placement, targeting areas of T2 abnormality, has also been described.[22]

Needle or catheter placement is typically confirmed by blood or lymph return. Contrast injection under fluoroscopy also allows for evaluation of the position of the needle tip, the communications between the different components of the malformation, and the local vascular anatomy, including the venous drainage. The volume of

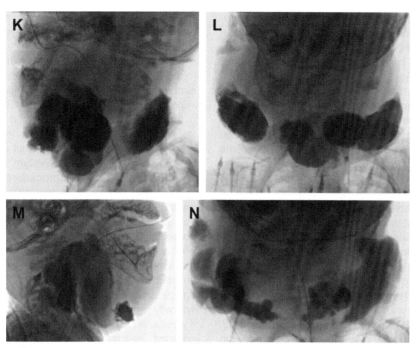

Fig. 7. (*continued*)

contrast injected intralesionally before opacification of the draining veins allows estimation of the volume of sclerosant needed. The initial contrast injection, in conjunction with the preoperative imaging (typically MR imaging), also allows for determination of what percentage of and what segments of the lesion will be accessible via the current injection.

A contrast agent, either water soluble, lipophilic (such as ethiodal), or negative contrast (air or carbon dioxide) is typically mixed with the sclerosant to allow fluoroscopic monitoring of the injection. In some practices, small and superficial vascular malformations are treated without fluoroscopic visualization, with pauses after what is felt to be an appropriate injection volume, and lesional thrombosis demonstrated by tissue induration within minutes of the injection. Intra-injection pallor or duskiness of the overlying skin is suggestive of skin irritation or ischemia, and the injection is stopped immediately, with cold sterile saline applied to the skin seeming to reduce the risk of blistering and ulceration.[23] Given the risks of extravasation, with consequent local soft tissue injury, or inadvertent embolization of sclerosant into the systemic venous drainage, with the potentially serious adverse effect described later in this article, we rarely perform sclerotherapy without image guidance. Once the predicted volume of needed sclerosant is approached, fluoroscopy typically reveals impending opacification of

adjacent normal venous drainage, and the injection is stopped. If the lesion, as assessed on the preoperative scans, has only been partially sclerosed, additional access is obtained with a second needle or cannula, and the process continued until the desired fraction of the lesion has been treated (Fig. 9E).

If venous drainage of the malformation is seen to be rapid on the initial contrast injection, the outflow must be slowed, typically with direct compression, either manually or via a device. After 2 to 3 minutes of pressure, the risk of systemic embolization is reduced, and the compression can be gradually relieved, under fluoroscopic visualization, if possible. Some have reported the use of a double needle technique, in which a second cannulation needle is introduced into the lesion before injection of sclerosant, to provide a low-pressure exit valve to allow external recovery of sclerosant during injection, reducing the risk of systemic misadministration.[24] Some head and neck malformations have venous drainage where the prospect of thrombosis or sclerosis is potentially perilous, such as lesions draining via the superior ophthalmic veins and cavernous sinuses or intracranially via a sinus pericranii. In these cases, where escape of sclerosant into the venous drainage could result in ophthalmic, cavernous, or intracranial venous thrombosis, scrupulous attention must be paid to compression of the lesional connection to the venous drainage. In cases where the connection is not superficial and therefore compression is not feasible, the communication must first be disrupted, either percutaneously or surgically, before sclerotherapy can be safely performed (Fig. 11).

Despite pretreatment with steroids, post-sclerotherapy edema can be significant, although it is usually of minimal clinical import. However, edema can present a serious problem in regions such as the orbit, where orbital compartment syndrome may result. The edema typically begins soon after sclerosant injection, reaches a maximum within 24 hours, and may last for up to 2 weeks. For orbit cases, we have ophthalmology colleagues on hand for potential decompression, if needed, following treatment. Moreover, we treat orbit vascular malformations only when symptomatic, ie, if there are visual changes or extraocular movement abnormalities. For complex lesions that partially involve the orbit, we target the extraorbital component, unless the patient has symptoms referable to the orbital component (see Fig. 10). Posttreatment edema in malformations involving the airway may result in inability to extubate the patient for several days. A pre-procedure otorhinolaryngology consult is routinely obtained for all of these patients, and the patients and anesthesia team are apprised of the likelihood of an extended ICU stay in advance.

Bleomycin, an antibiotic with cytotoxic properties, can be of particular use in orbit and airway patients, because of significantly less posttreatment edema. Multiple studies have demonstrated effective treatment of both venous and lymphatic malformations with bleomycin.[25] Nevertheless, the use of this agent has not found widespread acceptance in the United States because of concerns regarding its association with pulmonary fibrosis. However, it should be noted that this adverse effect has been described only at systemic doses that are much higher than those used in sclerotherapy, as is the case when bleomycin is used as a chemotherapeutic agent.[25]

Injection of sclerosant is typically painful, and given our pediatric patient base, the vast majority of our procedures are performed under general anesthesia. Sedation with ketamine can also be used for small lesions and short procedures.[23] Sclerosants cause immediate local hemolysis and subsequent hemoglobinuria. The latter is managed with generous hydration (doubling of the maintenance intravenous fluid for 4 hours postprocedure), monitoring of urinary output, and urinary alkalinization with sodium bicarbonate intravenous fluid. Patients with all but the very smallest lesions (who are administered only a few mL of sclerosant) have a Foley catheter

placed. The most serious systemic complications reported (particularly with the use of ethanol), including cardiovascular collapse, occur most often when sclerosing extensive extremity malformations. Given the much lower volumes of sclerosant typically used for treating head and neck lesions, such scenarios are fortunately rare.

After the procedure, antibiotic ointment is applied to puncture sites, and a loose dressing placed. Other than for the smallest of lesions, we typically monitor patients overnight in the hospital after the procedure. Postprocedure pain is typically mild to moderate (worse with ethanol), and most patients are given intravenous analgesics. Tapering doses of corticosteroids are given by some for 1 week. Elevation of the head of the bed and the use of ice packs can help reduce the swelling and discomfort. Other than for the smallest of lesions, most often multiple sessions are needed to achieve a satisfactory result; we typically space the sessions by approximately 6 weeks, and continue sclerosing so long as direct contrast injection demonstrates an accessible vascular or lymphatic space.

Despite the efficacy of combined interventional and surgical approaches, vascular malformations are often disfiguring and treatment is rarely curative. Coping with the life challenges posed by these lesions is an important goal for patients and their families, and psychologists and social workers play crucial roles on any vascular anomalies team.

Treatment of Venous Malformations

Localized pain from venous malformations is common, and often caused by focal thrombosis. In many cases, this can be effectively treated with daily aspirin (typically 81 mg), although efficacy varies. Coagulation of stagnant blood in ectatic channels triggers thrombin formation and the conversion of fibrinogen to fibrin, with subsequent fibrinolysis resulting in localized intravascular coagulopathy (LIC), seen in up to 42% of patients. This is associated with a rise in fibrin degradation products and a decrease in fibrinogen levels, with maintenance of normal prothrombin time and activated partial thromboplastin time.[26] In most cases, particularly for small lesions, LIC is well tolerated, although systemic activation of coagulation during surgical procedures can trigger disseminated intravascular coagulation (DIC). In patients with low fibrinogen levels, prophylactic treatment with subcutaneous low molecular weight heparin is initiated 10 days before the procedure, and continued for 10 to 14 days afterward; fibrinogen and D-dimer levels are typically followed.[26]

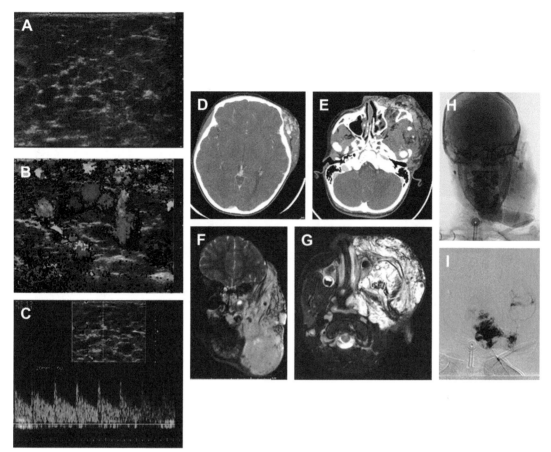

Fig. 8. (A) Characteristic spongiform appearance of venous malformation on gray-scale ultrasound. (B) Color Doppler interrogation reveals the compressible echolucent spaces to be vascular (venous). (C) Arterial signal is seen at the periphery of the lesion. (D, E) Contrast-enhanced axial CT images demonstrate irregular foci with avid enhancement, as well as phleboliths. Note the bony distortion of the left maxillary sinus and its frontal process. (F, G) Coronal and axial T2-weighted images demonstrate this massive venous malformation to be heterogeneous and trans-spatial. Phleboliths appear as rounded foci of hypointensity. (H) Unsubtracted fluoroscopic image demonstrates phleboliths as rounded radiopacities scattered throughout the soft tissue mass. (I) Surgical compartmentalization before sclerotherapy allowed for injection of sufficient sclerosant into well-defined regions of the large lesion to achieve a therapeutic concentration without reaching toxic dosage levels.

Generally, localized venous malformations have the best responses to sclerotherapy. Diffuse malformations are less likely to have a complete response, and the treatment should therefore be targeted at the most symptomatic portions; symptomatic improvement can often be excellent even in the absence of complete involution (see **Fig. 10**).

Venous malformations have been effectively treated with a variety of sclerosants. Absolute ethanol is perhaps the paradigmatic sclerosant, instantly precipitating endothelial proteins and inducing rapid thrombosis. Although some groups inject undiluted ethanol as a sclerosant without image guidance into low-flow vascular malformations, we always inject it under fluoroscopy, diluted 10:2 with ethiodol. Ethanol is the most

potent sclerosant agent and according to some has the lowest recurrence rate, but it suffers from the highest rate of serious complications.[23] These include both local adverse events, such as severe skin necrosis and local cranial nerve and peripheral nerve damage, and systemic effects, such as central nervous system depression, acute pulmonary hypertension, thromboembolism, DIC, hyperthermia, cardiac arrhythmias, and cardiovascular collapse and death. The risks, particularly the systemic risks, may be dose related, and the total dose should never exceed 1 mL/kg (with a maximum of 60 mL) per session. Some have suggested that systemic toxicity is related to the rate of systemic ethanol egress from the malformation rather than to absolute dose.[27] At doses

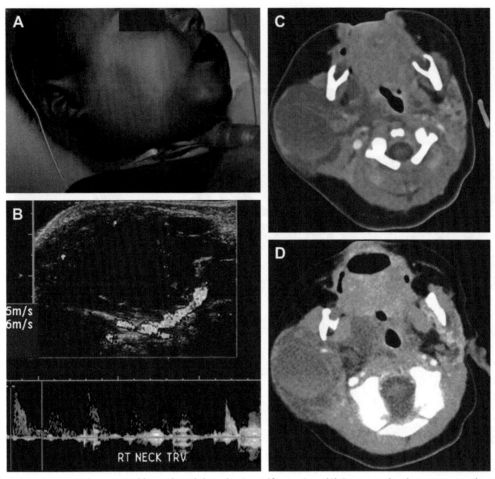

Fig. 9. (A) Right parotid space and lateral neck lymphatic malformation. (B) Sonography demonstrates character-istic macrocystic appearance, with a fluid-debris level. Vascularity is limited to septae and border zones of the lesion. (C) Pre-contrast axial CT demonstrates the right neck mass to be largely hypodense, with septations visible within the mass. (D) No significant enhancement of the macrocyst contents is seen with contrast administration. Some septal enhancement can be appreciated. (E) Multiple cannulas were used to sclerose the macrocyst until the opacified region approximated the macrocyst volume, as anticipated from the MR appearance. Axial pre-contrast (F, H) and post-contrast fat-suppressed images (G, I) on follow-up MR demonstrates regression of the macrocyst. Residual enhancing component with ill-defined borders is seen.

exceeding 0.75 mL/kg, the increase in systemic blood alcohol level is enough to invariably induce intoxication.[23] The risk of local soft tissue and cranial nerve injury from ethanol must be weighed carefully and may be unacceptable when the mal-formation involves vital structures, such as the facial nerve in parotid cases, or the orbital contents. Extravascular extravasation greatly increases the likelihood of nerve damage and skin necrosis. Reported morbidity rates vary wildly, and it is difficult to provide firm guidance to patients. However, clearly ethanol should be used only by experienced practitioners who have excellent anesthesia and ICU support.

Given the potential morbidity of ethanol, we prefer to use detergent agents for sclerosis of

head and neck venous malformations. These agents have both a proven safety profile and good efficacy. The agents include sodium tetra-decyl sulfate (STS, our preferred agent, approved by the Food and Drug Administration for the treat-ment of varicose veins), polydocanol, sodium morrhuate,[28] and ethanolamine. Reported compli-cations are both milder and more infrequent relative to ethanol, with only one report of cardiovascular collapse from detergents (polydocanol).

Detergent agents can be mixed with either water-soluble or oily contrast agents, such as ethiodal. Foaming of detergents has been re-ported to increase efficacy.[29,30] It is speculated that this may relate to the increased surface area for contact between the endothelium and the

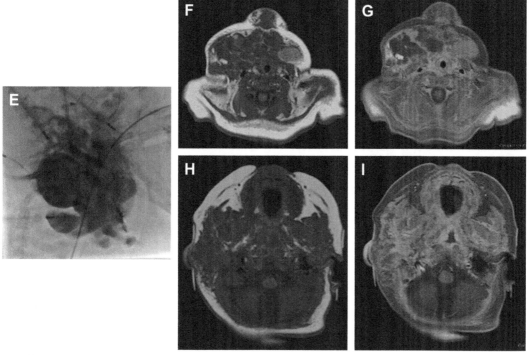

Fig. 9. (*continued*)

sclerosant microbubbles, as opposed to the liquid form of the agent. Foaming can be achieved by intermixing 10 mL of sodium tetradecyl sulfate 3% with 2 mL of ethiodol and 10 mL of air via a three-way stopcock, with brisk back-and-forth injection between two syringes.

As mentioned previously, bleomycin has been used widely outside the United States for the treatment of venous malformations,[25] and is reported to induce little postprocedure edema. Theoretically, bleomycin has the potential risk of systemic toxicities associated with its use as a chemotherapeutic agent, including pulmonary fibrosis, alopecia, and skin pigmentation. However, the doses typically used in sclerotherapy are well below the maximal systemic limit of 0.5 mg/kg, and such complications have never been reported as a result of sclerotherapy.

In cases of large venous varices, platinum coils (bare or fibered) may be useful as adjuncts to sclerotherapy, where direct sclerosant injection would be ineffective or dangerous. Coils can be deployed percutaneously through a micropuncture sheath or large cannula. In rare cases of rapid venous drainage, where preservation of normal venous drainage is desired, a catheter can be advanced through the malformation to its junction with normal veins, where coils can be deployed to occlude the anastomosis. Sclerosant can then be safely injected into the malformation.[23]

An additional adjunct to sclerotherapy consists of percutaneously injecting a liquid polymer. These agents were designed for the treatment of high-flow vascular malformations (see our companion chapter in this volume), do not cause any significant sclerosing effect, and typically do not induce the kind of avid edema caused by sclerosants. There is little mid- to long-term efficacy data on the older of the liquid polymers (N-butyl-cyanoacrylate, NBCA) for the treatment of venous malformations, but it can be very effective in the preoperative setting, where only short-term occlusion is needed. The newer of these liquid agents, ethylene vinyl alcohol copolymer (Onyx, EV3 Neurovascular, Irvine, CA), is injected in very deliberate fashion, and through the use of strategic injection strategies, can be directed toward specific targets within the lesion. This may offer an alternative means for occluding lesional anastomoses with normal venous outflow that must be preserved, such as the superior ophthalmic veins or sinus pericranii, allowing for the safe injection of sclerosant to follow (see **Fig. 11**). n-BCA can be used in similar fashion.

Treatment of Lymphatic Malformations

An overarching principle here is that macrocystic lymphatic malformations typically show excellent response to sclerotherapy, whereas microcystic

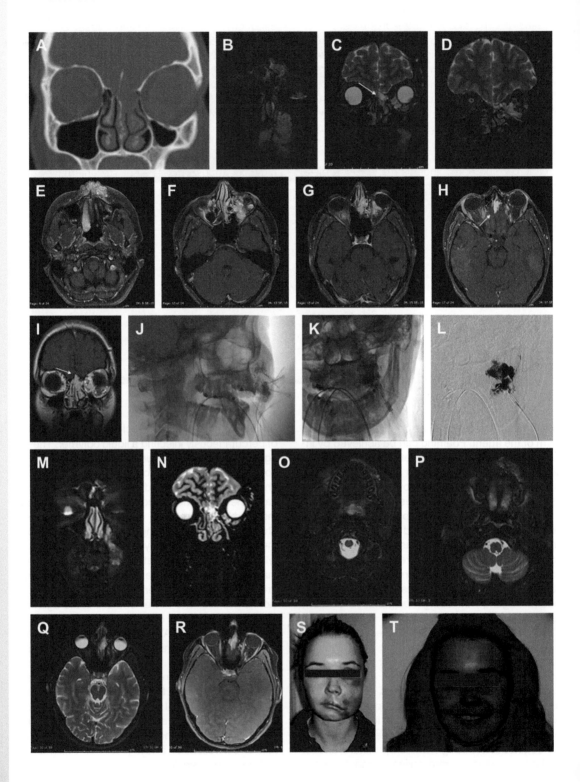

lymphatic malformations are both technically difficult to treat and tend to show a poor response.[31] For microcystic lesions, conservative management is recommended, with surgery considered for cosmetic and functional considerations.[11] Radiofrequency ablation has also been reported.[32,33]

Sclerosants used for treating macrocystic lymphatic malformations include ethanol, doxycycline, bleomycin, Ethibloc, and OK-432. The latter two are not approved for use in the United States, although OK-432 is being studied in an American multicenter trial. We prefer doxycycline (Doxy 100, APP Pharmaceuticals, Schaumburg, IL), at a concentration of 10 mg/mL, for most lymphatic malformations because of its very low morbidity rate (including a low incidence of postprocedure edema) and its efficacy. Bleomycin is similarly effective for macrocystic LM and also tends to induce little postprocedure edema. As mentioned earlier, the systemic toxicities associated with bleomycin use as a chemotherapeutic agent have never been reported as a result of sclerotherapy. Ethanol is certainly effective for localized macrocystic LM, but as mentioned above, carries a higher risk of tissue and cranial nerve damage, along with expected significant postprocedure edema.

OK-432, consisting of a solution of killed streptococci group A in a penicillin suspension, has been used successfully in Europe and Japan. It induces an inflammatory reaction with resultant scarring, and has minimal side effects. It has been used for treating both lymphatic and venous malformations, with good results.

Sclerotherapy technique for LM slightly differs from that for VM. Individual cysts are cannulated under ultrasound guidance. For most lesions this is done with angiocatheters, but for large cysts a pigtail catheter can be introduced (**Fig. 6**G). The fluid contents are aspirated and the volume noted, and the cyst is then injected with the sclerosant of choice. For very large cysts, the catheter is often secured in place, injecting and draining cysts sequentially for several days.

Because of the higher risk of infection for lymphatic malformations, we treat patients with prophylactic antibiotics during sclerotherapy; many practitioners continue prophylactic antibiotic administration for 7 to 10 days. Cyst involution can be assessed approximately 6 weeks after the procedure. We typically schedule needed additional sessions approximately at 6- to 8-week intervals.

CHALLENGES INVOLVING PARTICULAR HEAD AND NECK LOCATIONS
Orbital Vascular Malformations

Orbital vascular malformations present a particular challenge because of potentially devastating orbital compartment syndrome from postprocedure edema. The margin of error for needle placement and sclerosant control is small. Although most cases are done with ultrasound guidance for needle placement through the upper or lower lid, some have used CT and MR image fusion and frameless stereotactic guidance for needle placement[34] for ethanol injection. Some authors advise against the use of ethanol in the orbit. Intraoperative injection of N-butyl-2-cyanoacrylate (which, as mentioned earlier, does not elicit an avid inflammatory reaction) into an orbital VM immediately before resection has been reported. Some have suggested that sclerotherapy should be avoided altogether for orbital venous malformations, given the risk of orbital compartment syndrome and blindness.

Orbital venous malformations may be quiescent for years, but orbital lymphatic malformations are

Fig. 10. Venous malformation involving the upper lip, cheek, left orbit, and nasal cavity, with intracranial extension. The patient's clinical complaint was oral bleeding and episodic left facial pain. There was a mild degree of proptosis. (A) Coronal thin-cut CT demonstrates dehiscence of the cribriform plate. (B–D) Coronal T2-weighted images with fat suppression demonstrate the hyperintense venous malformation to involve the left upper lip, cheek, and left inferomedial orbit. Hyperintensity immediately inferior to the left gyrus rectus (*arrow* in C) represents VM extending through the dehiscent cribriform plate. Axial (E–H) and coronal (I) post-contrast T1-weighted images with fat suppression demonstrate avid enhancement of the T2-hyperintense tissue, consistent with venous malformation. The intracranial component is denoted by the arrow in H and I. (J, K) Unsubtracted and (L) subtracted fluoroscopic images demonstrate that sclerotherapy was directed to the inferior compartment of the lesion, in the lip. Contrast injection demonstrated no appreciable runoff toward the orbital and nasal compartments. At least on theoretical grounds, injection of the sclerosant into the intracranial compartment, with its ensuing edema, could be precarious. Coronal (M, N) and axial (O–Q) T2-weighted images demonstrate significant regression of the lip and cheek component of the venous malformation after treatment. (R) Post-contrast axial T1-weighted image with fat suppression demonstrates regression of the intraorbital component. Although only the lip was injected with sclerosant (J–L), posttreatment edema was seen in the cheek and infraorbital region as well (S). After two sessions of sclerotherapy, the facial pain was markedly improved, there were no further bleeding episodes, and there was an excellent cosmetic response to treatment (T).

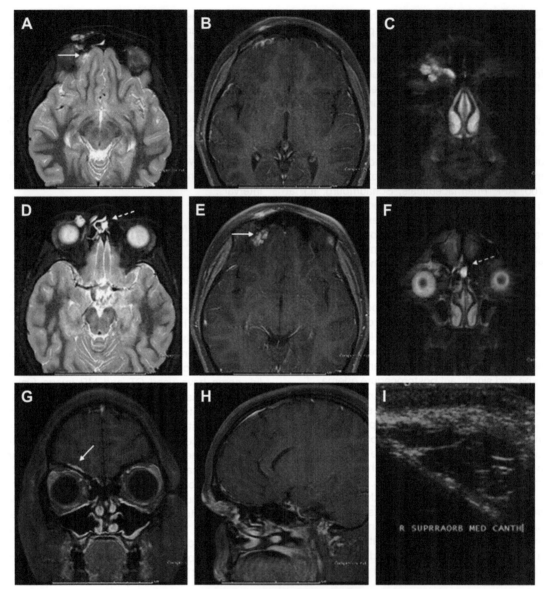

Fig. 11. Axial T2 (*A, D*) and post-contrast, fat-suppressed (*B, E*) images demonstrate a supraorbital T2-hyperintense lesion with avid enhancement that extends intracranially (*solid arrows*) as well as into the ethmoid air cells (*dashed arrows*). The lesion extent is appreciated on coronal (*C, F, G*) and oblique sagittal (*H*) images as well. Sonography (*I*) demonstrates the spongiform appearance characteristic of venous malformation. The patient presented with catamenial right retro-orbital headache and copious epistaxis, likely from hormone sensitivity of the venous malformation. Frontal and lateral unsubtracted views of the percutaneous contrast injection (*J, K*). Lateral subtracted view (*L*) demonstrates rapid contrast drainage from the lesion via the superior ophthalmic vein and cavernous sinus. Injection of sclerosant in this setting could elicit venous and sinus thrombosis. (*M, N*) Frontal and lateral unsubtracted views demonstrating an onyx cast, injected percutaneously. Control over onyx flow allowed injection to proceed just to the junction point between the venous malformation and the superior ophthalmic vein (*dashed arrow*). Lateral (*O*) and frontal (*P*) subtracted fluoroscopic images demonstrate nonopacification of the superior ophthalmic vein/cavernous system, with all drainage now via lateral facial veins. Sclerosant could then be safely injected, resulting in complete resolution of the clinical symptoms.

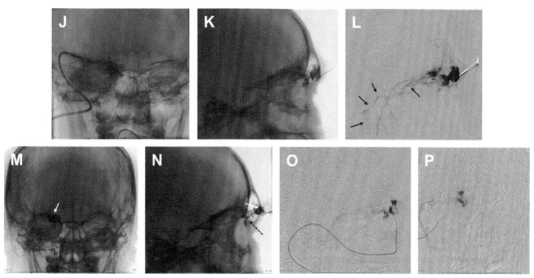

Fig. 11. (*continued*)

rarely silent lesions. A recent report[35] described that over half the patients with periorbital lymphatic malformations had intralesional bleeding, over a quarter had infections, three quarters had intermittent swelling, approximately half had proptosis, and 20% had pain. Forty percent of the patients had diminished vision, and 7% eventually lost their sight in the affected eye. Most patients required multiple treatment sessions, which included sclerotherapy in 40% and resection in 57%.

A recent retrospective study of patients with orbital lymphatic or venolymphatic malformations by the same group[36] found that over two thirds had an associated intracranial vascular anomaly. Their recommendation was to include intracranial imaging in the workup of orbital vascular anomalies (Fig. 12).

Airway Vascular Malformations

Given the expected posttreatment edema after sclerotherapy, the ability to extubate the patient safely may be precluded for several days. Patients with airway vascular malformations often are complex intubation and extubation cases, and the team should be prepared for potential fiberoptic–guided intubation or even tracheostomy, should the need arise. Airway devices such as laryngeal mask airway, nasal trumpets, and others, should be available. The head of the bed is ideally kept somewhat elevated to promote venous drainage, and coughing and bucking should be minimized.

Published reports on management of airway low-flow vascular malformations are few. Clinical presentation may involve stridor (particularly in a small infant airway further narrowed by a malformation), sleep apnea, or dysphagia. Ohlms and colleagues[37] recommended a combination of sclerotherapy and laser photocoagulation delivered by direct laryngoscopy when needed, with multiple treatments and careful long-term follow-up required. Despite optimized treatment, some patients with airway malformations will require tracheostomy, and patients with large malformations occasionally have a tracheostomy placed prophylactically before the first sclerotherapy session.

OUTCOME/COMPLICATIONS

It is important that patients and their families understand that interventional treatment of slow-flow vascular malformations has inherent risk, although it is difficult to quantify the risk confidently, as reported rates vary tremendously.[24] Burrows and Mason[23] reported an overall complication rate of 12% for sclerotherapy procedures to treat venous malformations. The risk of peripheral neuropathy is cited as approximately 1%, and this for the most part is transient. Skin blistering is common and typically heals uneventfully. Skin necrosis with permanent scarring is reported to occur in 10% to 15% of cases; the risk is highest where the malformation itself has a superficial component that involves the skin. For lesions involving the tongue, buccal surfaces, soft palate, or airway, marked postprocedural edema can cause transient dysphagia. If sclerosant directly infiltrates muscle tissue, atrophy and contracture may result.[38]

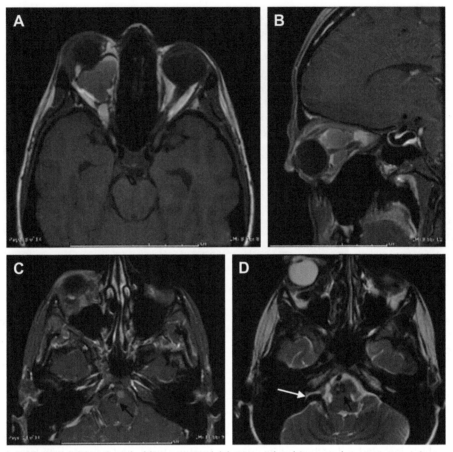

Fig. 12. Post-contrast axial (*A, C*) and oblique sagittal (*B*) T1-weighted images demonstrate an intraconal post-septal macrocystic lymphatic malformation. Fluid-fluid levels can be appreciated. T2-weighted image through the skull base demonstrates a round heterogeneous lesion in the lower pons with a hypointense rim characteristic of cerebral cavernous malformation (*black arrow*). An associated developmental venous anomaly (*white arrow*) is present. The patient was developing diplopia and diminished extraocular movements, but when she presented for sclerotherapy, the malformation had auto-decompressed and treatment was deferred.

Prognosis of sclerotherapy for macrocystic lymphatic malformations is generally excellent, with some degree of improvement seen in almost all cases.[25,31] In a systematic review comparing various sclerosants for LM,[39] OK-432 was found to have 43% complete response, 24% good response, 17% fair/poor response, and 15% no response. Bleomycin was found to have a 35% complete response, 37% good response, 18% fair/poor response, and 12% no response. Doxy-cycline sclerotherapy was recently reported to result in complete clinical resolution in 100% of cases for macrocystic lesions, with over 90% radiographic resolution.[40] A recent prospective study of foamed detergent sclerotherapy treatment for venous malformations reported that at 6-month follow-up, 45% of patients had no recanalization and another 45% had partial

recanalization. Sessions were repeated until patient satisfaction was achieved or little improvement was seen from continued treatment.[29] Most treatment-response studies have used patient questionnaires for assessment, inquiring about both symptomatic and cosmetic improvement. Attempts to use imaging follow-up have resulted in the finding that imaging improvement does not necessarily correlate with symptomatic relief. As expected, treatment response for diffuse lesions is significantly poorer than for focal lesions.

SUMMARY

Low-flow vascular malformations represent errors in normal development involving the venous, lymphatic, and capillary systems. Patients present because of pain, cosmetic concerns, or because of symptoms related to mass effect of the malformation on vital structures. The latter is particularly true in the head and neck, given the concentration of vital structures in very contained anatomic regions. Our approach to workup and treatment is intrinsically multidisciplinary, with interventional, neurointerventional, surgical, and, increasingly, medical arms, as well as the vital involvement of professional support for the psychological and social issues that arise. Despite the complexity and rarity of these types of cases, most patients can be significantly helped through this kind of multifaceted intervention.

ACKNOWLEDGMENTS

The authors express their profound indebtedness to the physicians and staff of the Vascular Anomalies Center at Children's Hospital Boston, headed by Drs. John B. Mulliken and Stephen J. Fishman, without whom this work would not have been possible. Additionally, the authors thank the staff of the Interventional Radiology Division at Children's Hospital Boston and the Neurointerventional Service at Brigham and Women's Hospital.

REFERENCES

1. Mulliken JB, Glowacki J. Hemangiomas and vascular malformations in infants and children: a classification based on endothelial characteristics. Plast Reconstr Surg 1982;69:412–22.
2. Selim MM, Kelly KM, Nelson JS, et al. Confocal microscopy study of nerves and blood vessels in untreated and treated port wine stains: preliminary observations. Dermatol Surg 2004;30:892–7.
3. Jacobs AH, Walton RG. The incidence of birthmarks in the neonate. Pediatrics 1976;58:218–22.
4. Garzon MC, Huang JT, Enjolras O, et al. Vascular malformations: part I. J Am Acad Dermatol 2007; 56:353–70 quiz 371–4.
5. Tallman B, Tan OT, Morelli JG, et al. Location of port-wine stains and the likelihood of ophthalmic and/or central nervous system complications. Pediatrics 1991;87:323–7.
6. Hennedige AA, Quaba AA, Al-Nakib K. Sturge-Weber syndrome and dermatomal facial port-wine stains: incidence, association with glaucoma, and pulsed tunable dye laser treatment effectiveness. Plast Reconstr Surg 2008;121:1173–80.
7. Eerola I, Boon LM, Mulliken JB, et al. Capillary malformation-arteriovenous malformation, a new clinical and genetic disorder caused by RASA1 mutations. Am J Hum Genet 2003;73:1240–9.
8. Frech M, John J, Pizon V, et al. Inhibition of GTPase activating protein stimulation of Ras-p21 GTPase by the Krev-1 gene product. Science 1990;249:169–71.
9. Katugampola GA, Lanigan SW. Five years' experience of treating port wine stains with the flashlamp-pumped pulsed dye laser. Br J Dermatol 1997;137:750–4.
10. Boon LM, Mulliken JB, Vikkula M, et al. Assignment of a locus for dominantly inherited venous malformations to chromosome 9p. Hum Mol Genet 1994;3:1583–7.
11. Dubois J, Garel L. Imaging and therapeutic approach of hemangiomas and vascular malformations in the pediatric age group. Pediatr Radiol 1999;29:879–93.
12. Boon LM, Mulliken JB, Enjolras O, et al. Glomuvenous malformation (glomangioma) and venous malformation: distinct clinicopathologic and genetic entities. Arch Dermatol 2004;140:971–6.
13. Garzon MC, Huang JT, Enjolras O, et al. Vascular malformations. Part II: associated syndromes. J Am Acad Dermatol 2007;56:541–64.
14. Perkins JA, Maniglia C, Magit A, et al. Clinical and radiographic findings in children with spontaneous lymphatic malformation regression. Otolaryngol Head Neck Surg 2008;138:772–7.
15. Smith RJ. Lymphatic malformations. Lymphat Res Biol 2004;2:25–31.
16. Padwa BL, Hayward PG, Ferraro NF, et al. Cervicofacial lymphatic malformation: clinical course, surgical intervention, and pathogenesis of skeletal hypertrophy. Plast Reconstr Surg 1995;95:951–60.
17. Konez O, Burrows PE. Magnetic resonance of vascular anomalies. Magn Reson Imaging Clin N Am 2002;10:363–88, vii.
18. Rifenburg NE, Batton B, Vade A. Ruptured retroperitoneal lymphatic malformation. Comput Med Imaging Graph 2006;30:61–3.
19. Donnelly LF, Adams DM, Bisset GS 3rd. Vascular malformations and hemangiomas: a practical approach in a multidisciplinary clinic. AJR Am J Roentgenol 2000;174:597–608.
20. Jackson IT, Keskin M, Yavuzer R, et al. Compartmentalization of massive vascular malformations. Plast Reconstr Surg 2005;115:10–21.
21. Donnelly LF, Bissett GS 3rd, Adams DM. Combined sonographic and fluoroscopic guidance: a modified technique for percutaneous sclerosis of low-flow vascular malformations. AJR Am J Roentgenol 1999;173:655–7.
22. Nanz D, Andreisek G, Frohlich JM, et al. Contrast material-enhanced visualization of the ablation medium for magnetic resonance-monitored ethanol injection therapy: imaging and safety aspects. J Vasc Interv Radiol 2006;17:95–102.
23. Burrows PE, Mason KP. Percutaneous treatment of low flow vascular malformations. J Vasc Interv Radiol 2004;15:431–45.
24. Puig S, Casati B, Staudenherz A, et al. Vascular low-flow malformations in children: current concepts for classification, diagnosis and therapy. Eur J Radiol 2005;53:35–45.

25. Muir T, Kirsten M, Fourie P, et al. Intralesional bleomycin injection (IBI) treatment for haemangiomas and congenital vascular malformations. Pediatr Surg Int 2004;19:766–73.

26. Dompmartin A, Acher A, Thibon P, et al. Association of localized intravascular coagulopathy with venous malformations. Arch Dermatol 2008;144:873–7.

27. Wong GA, Armstrong DC, Robertson JM. Cardiovascular collapse during ethanol sclerotherapy in a pediatric patient. Paediatr Anaesth 2006;16:343–6.

28. Yildirim I, Cinar C, Aydin Y, et al. Sclerotherapy to a large cervicofacial vascular malformation: a case report with 24 years' follow-up. Head Neck 2005; 27:639–43.

29. Yamaki T, Nozaki M, Sakurai H, et al. Prospective randomized efficacy of ultrasound-guided foam sclerotherapy compared with ultrasound-guided liquid sclerotherapy in the treatment of symptomatic venous malformations. J Vasc Surg 2008;47:578–84.

30. Hamel-Desnos C, Desnos P, Wollmann JC, et al. Evaluation of the efficacy of polidocanol in the form of foam compared with liquid form in sclerotherapy of the greater saphenous vein: initial results. Dermatol Surg 2003;29:1170–5 [discussion 1175].

31. Alomari AI, Karian VE, Lord DJ, et al. Percutaneous sclerotherapy for lymphatic malformations: a retrospective analysis of patient-evaluated improvement. J Vasc Interv Radiol 2006;17:1639–48.

32. Grimmer JF, Mulliken JB, Burrows PE, et al. Radiofrequency ablation of microcystic lymphatic malformation in the oral cavity. Arch Otolaryngol Head Neck Surg 2006;132:1251–6.

33. van der Linden E, Overbosch J, Kroft LJ. Radiofrequency ablation for treatment of symptomatic low-flow vascular malformations after previous unsuccessful therapy. J Vasc Interv Radiol 2005; 16:747–50.

34. Ernemann U, Westendorff C, Troitzsch D, et al. Navigation-assisted sclerotherapy of orbital venolymphatic malformation: a new guidance technique for percutaneous treatment of low-flow vascular malformations. AJNR Am J Neuroradiol 2004;25:1792–5.

35. Greene AK, Burrows PE, Smith L, et al. Periorbital lymphatic malformation: clinical course and management in 42 patients. Plast Reconstr Surg 2005;115:22–30.

36. Bisdorff A, Mulliken JB, Carrico J, et al. Intracranial vascular anomalies in patients with periorbital lymphatic and lymphaticovenous malformations. AJNR Am J Neuroradiol 2007;28:335–41.

37. Ohlms LA, Forsen J, Burrows PE. Venous malformation of the pediatric airway. Int J Pediatr Otorhinolaryngol 1996;37:99–114.

38. Smithers CJ, Vogel AM, Kozakewich HP, et al. An injectable tissue-engineered embolus prevents luminal recanalization after vascular sclerotherapy. J Pediatr Surg 2005;40:920–5.

39. Acevedo JL, Shah RK, Brietzke SE. Nonsurgical therapies for lymphangiomas: a systematic review. Otolaryngol Head Neck Surg 2008;138:418–24.

40. Nehra D, Jacobson L, Barnes P, et al. Doxycycline sclerotherapy as primary treatment of head and neck lymphatic malformations in children. J Pediatr Surg 2008;43:451–60.

Neurointerventional Management of High-Flow Vascular Malformations of the Head and Neck

Isaac C. Wu, MD[a], Darren B. Orbach, MD, PhD[b],*

KEYWORDS

- High-flow vascular malformation
- Arteriovenous malformation (AVM)
- Arteriovenous fistula (AVF) • Embolization
- Syndromic vascular anomalies

Vascular malformations of the head and neck are rare lesions, thought to result from errors in vascular morphogenesis. These lesions can be subdivided either histologically based on the predominant vascular channel type, or functionally based on the flow characteristics, ie, high-flow versus low-flow lesions.[1]

Our focus is on the high-flow vascular malformations (HFVMs) of the head and neck, largely arteriovenous malformations (AVM), and arteriovenous fistulae (AVF). Other vascular lesions with high-flow characteristics, such as infantile hemangiomas during their proliferative stage and other vascular tumors, are outside our purview; these other lesions have natural histories and treatment paradigms that fundamentally differ from the vascular malformations we consider here.

The high-flow lesions have arteriovenous shunting as an intrinsic feature, ie, shunting of blood under arterial pressure and arterial flow rates into the venous system; herein is the root of much of the pathophysiology of these lesions. The AV shunt presents a risk of hemorrhage, most commonly from rupture of venous structures not designed for arterial pressure, although arterial rupture, particularly at weak points such as flow-related or intranidal aneurysms, certainly occurs as well. Additionally, the AV shunt likely causes a localized steal phenomenon, with chronically ischemic tissue in the vicinity of the AVM leading to pain, infection, skin and mucosal breakdown, and so forth.

The morphology of the shunt can take two forms: (1) a fistula, or a direct communication from an artery of visible caliber into a vein of visible caliber, or (2) a nidus, a network of abnormal vascular channels bridging the feeding arteries and draining veins. In either case, normal arterioles and the capillary bed are absent.[2–4] AVMs and fistulae are not mutually exclusive, as it is not uncommon to see fistulous foci within a complex AVM nidus. Compared with the low-flow vascular lesions of the head and neck reviewed elsewhere in this issue, the HFVMs are rare.[5] The rarity of these lesions and the complexity of the pathophysiology pose a significant management challenge, and no standard treatment paradigm has been established.

[a] Neuroradiology Division, Brigham and Women's Hospital, Harvard Medical School, 75 Francis Street, PBB 356, Boston, MA 02115, USA
[b] Neurointerventional Radiology, Children's Hospital Boston, Brigham and Women's Hospital, Harvard Medical School, 75 Francis Street, PBB 356, Boston, MA 02115, USA
* Corresponding author.
E-mail address: dorbach@partners.org (D.B. Orbach).

Neuroimag Clin N Am 19 (2009) 219–240
doi:10.1016/j.nic.2009.01.005
1052-5149/09/$ – see front matter © 2009 Elsevier Inc. All rights reserved.

Proposed treatment algorithms, however, usually involve sclerotherapy, endovascular or percutaneous embolization, surgical excision, or some combination of these modalities.[2,5–7] In this article, we focus on the endovascular treatments for various HFVMs (mainly AVMs) of the head and neck, as proposed in the literature, and elaborate on our approach to these lesions. By way of definition, by "sclerotherapy" we refer to the injection of an agent designed to ultimately convert a vascular space into a scar, typically by inducing a cascade of inflammation and thrombosis. Sclerosants are almost always injected percutaneously or transmucosally (as described elsewhere in this issue), although transarterial injection of absolute ethanol would be an example of intravascular sclerotherapy. By "embolization," we refer to the injection or deployment of a largely inert substance designed to impede flow or passively fill a vascular space. Examples of liquid embolics include n-butyl cyanoacrylate (n-BCA) and Onyx, whereas examples of solid embolics include polyvinyl alcohol particles (PVA) and coils.

INCIDENCE AND CLINICAL PRESENTATION

The pathogenesis of vascular malformations is complex and incompletely understood. Postulated mechanisms have been summarized in several recent reviews.[2,3] Rather than representing neoplasms, these lesions result from errors in vascular development.

HFVMs of the head and neck are quite rare and their true incidence is unknown. There may be a slightly higher prevalence in girls, with at least one series reporting a female-to-male ratio of 1.5:1.[5] The lesions are likely present at birth, but many are not clinically evident until later in life. Although clinical presentation is most common between late infancy and early school age, the potential age of presentation varies from the neonatal period to middle age. HFVMs usually enlarge in proportion with the growth of the child, but rapid progression can be provoked by hormonal changes (eg, puberty, pregnancy) or trauma (eg, direct force, surgical intervention, infection, thrombosis). The associated signs and symptoms are largely dependent upon the extent of the lesion and the site of involvement in the head and neck.[5]

The most common site for AVMs in the head and neck is the cheek (31%), followed by the ear (16%) and the nose (11%), whereas areas such as the mandible (5%) and maxilla (4%) are less commonly involved.[5] Traditionally, the Schobinger staging system has been used to assess AVMs. In stage I, the lesions are quiescent and asymptomatic. In stage II, the lesions demonstrate expansion but remain largely asymptomatic. Overlying skin changes, increased local temperature, or palpable pulse and thrill are often present. In stage III, the lesions become symptomatic, most commonly with pain, ulceration, and hemorrhage. In stage IV, a high degree of AV shunting leads to cardiac decompensation. Despite its widespread use, it is debatable how valuable the Schobinger classification is in the head and neck—extracranial lesions are virtually never large enough to cause cardiac overload, the natural history is most often unpredictable rather than progressing neatly from stage to stage,[5] and the decision to treat or not at a given point is not a strict function of the Schobinger stage.[4,5] A treatment dilemma often occurs with the stage I lesions, which may remain stable for a long period of time. At this juncture, there is no convincing evidence that intervening early alters the natural history of HFVMs, and our practice is to typically closely follow stage I lesions expectantly, and delay treatment attempts until rapid progression (stage II) or complications (stage III) become evident.[4] However, faced with a giant, difficult-to-manage AVM in a teenager or young adult, one cannot help but wonder retrospectively whether earlier intervention would have led to different clinical evolution.

DIAGNOSIS

The diagnosis of a high-flow vascular malformation can be reliably made based on clinical history and physical exam. On exam, the high-flow lesions are usually reddish, warm, firm, and pulsatile (Fig. 1). Local skin ischemia, ulceration, and/or hemorrhage are frequently seen with more advanced lesions (Fig. 2). As described elsewhere in this issue, these are not typical features for low-flow lesions,[1] and as such, the diagnosis is usually not dependent upon imaging results.

Cross-sectional imaging, including computerized tomographic angiography and magnetic resonance angiography, can be valuable in delineating the tissue spaces involved by the AVM and its

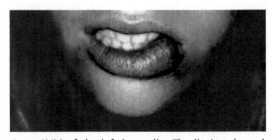

Fig. 1. AVM of the left lower lip. The lip is enlarged, warm, reddish, and pulsatile to the touch.

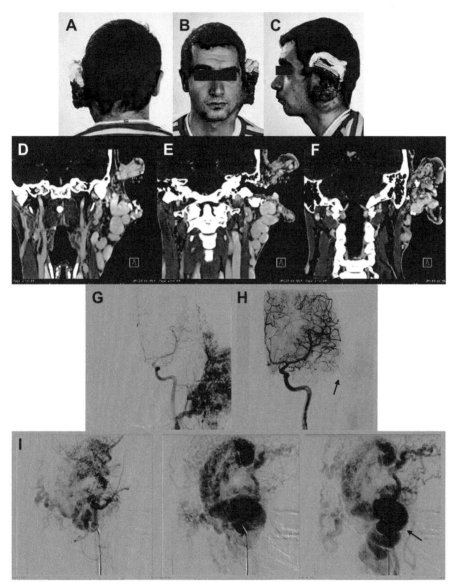

Fig. 2. (A) Giant AVM of the left ear and lateral neck. The AVM was quiescent during early childhood and began to grow and cause pain during puberty. After attempted embolization with n-BCA there was explosive growth of the AVM, with necrosis, chronic infection, and daily bleeding from the left ear. (B, C) Much of the bulk of the mass in the left neck resulted from the ectatic venous pouches inferomedial to the ear, as seen on the coronal computerized tomographic angiography images (D–F). Frontal angiographic views of a left common carotid (G) and internal carotid (H) injection. Note the preferential runoff to the AVM, resulting in poor opacification of the ICA in (G). The extracranial AVM has recruited a pial MCA branch, which crosses the calvarium to provide collateral supply (arrow in H). This branch will regress with direct treatment of the AVM. (I) Lateral angiographic views of a left external carotid injection demonstrating rapid arteriovenous shunting via a diffuse nidus, with drainage via the ectatic veins seen earlier (black arrow in K). The main arterial supply is via the superficial temporal and posterior auricular arteries. Lateral (J) and frontal (K) angiographic views of a left vertebral artery injection, demonstrating collateral supply to the AVM via reconstitution of the left occipital artery (white arrows). Unsubtracted fluoroscopic views of the Onyx cast, in lateral (L) and frontal (M) projections. Lateral (N) and frontal (O) angiographic views of a left external carotid injection post-embolization demonstrates nonopacification of much of the AVM. The draining veins have diminished in size but are still prominently seen in O. However, embolization has converted this to a surgically manageable lesion (P). Residual prominence of the ectatic veins in the neck has continued to shrink in the interval since surgery.

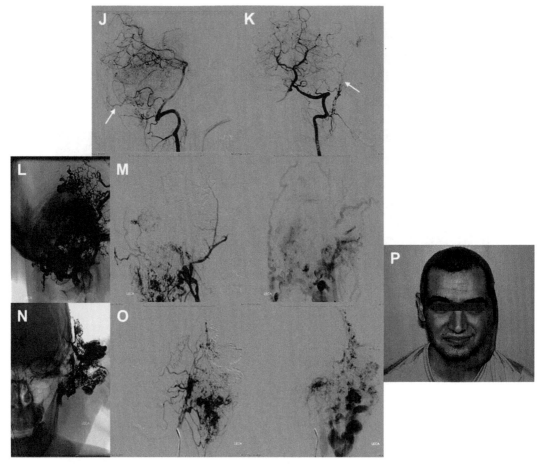

Fig. 2. (*continued*)

effect on adjacent structures. However, catheter angiography continues to provide the highest spatial resolution available, as well as critical insight into the dynamics of flow in the lesion. The selection of images in this article reflects our bias in this regard.

For noninvasive cross-sectional imaging workup of HFVMs, magnetic resonance imaging (MR imaging) is the modality of choice because of its superior soft tissue contrast and ability to display the extent of the lesion. On MR imaging, HFVMs characteristically show dilated feeding arteries and draining veins with flow voids on T2-weighted imaging and corresponding hyperintense signal on flow-enhanced gradient-echo sequences. The nidus of an AVM may be delineated as smaller caliber curvilinear abnormalities, although often the extent of the nidus visualized by catheter angiography is significantly underestimated on MR. Newer sequences, such as time-resolved MR angiography and MR perfusion imaging, may further characterize the flow characteristics and hemodynamics.[8,9] Computed tomography (CT) is crucial in delineating skeletal involvement, in particular the mandible, skull base, orbits, and calvarium. Color Doppler ultrasonography, portable and widely available, is helpful in verifying high-flow vascularity if the initial diagnosis is in doubt, and can accurately delineate the extent of the lesion, although this mainly holds for small superficial cases.[10]

THERAPEUTIC GOAL AND ENDOVASCULAR MANAGEMENT

Although lethal complications such as massive hemorrhage do occur, HFVMs of the head and neck are usually not life-threatening. Given the inherently trans-spatial nature of these lesions, the therapeutic goal for most patients with complex lesions is symptomatic control, preservation of vital functions (eg, vision, hearing, or mastication), or aesthetic restoration, rather than a complete "cure." Treatment options may depend on the site, size, and complexity of the lesion, as well as the experience and preference of the treating physicians. The available treatment modalities include percutaneous or endovascular embolization or sclerotherapy and surgical resection. A multidisciplinary approach is essential.

Some authors have advocated sclerotherapy as the initial treatment modality when the AVM

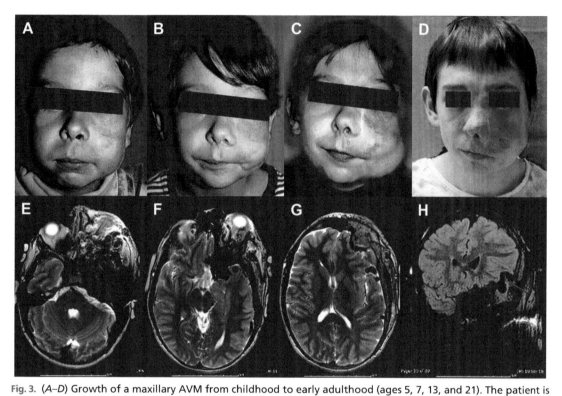

Fig. 3. (A–D) Growth of a maxillary AVM from childhood to early adulthood (ages 5, 7, 13, and 21). The patient is status post multiple sessions of embolization with alcohol, with a partial maxillectomy and attempted resection at age 6. There has been progressive proptosis and loss of vision and extraocular mobility of the left eye. The patient has had nearly daily epistaxis since childhood, but began having copious bleeding at age 21, with several life-threatening hemorrhages requiring large transfusions. (E–G) Axial T2-weighted images demonstrating infiltration of the AVM nidus and associated flow-voids into the entirety of the left orbit, as well as intracranially. Large flow void over the lateral temporal lobe, well demonstrated on the coronal FLAIR image (arrow in H), represents a main intracranial venous drainage pathway for this extracranial AVM. The risk of intracranial hemorrhage from an extracranial AVM with intracranial extension such as this is unknown. Lateral (I) and frontal (J) angiographic views of a right internal carotid artery injection demonstrate recruitment of mandibular (black arrows) and cavernous (white arrow) branches of the ICA to supply the AVM. Lateral (K) and frontal (L) angiographic views of a left internal carotid injection demonstrate a massively ectatic left ophthalmic artery (dashed black arrow). Note the paucity of intracranial runoff by comparison with the ophthalmic runoff. Dashed white arrow demonstrates the large left temporal cortical vein draining the AVM toward the sigmoid sinus. Frontal (M, O) and lateral (N, P) unsubtracted fluoroscopic images demonstrating progressive embolization, with growth of the Onyx cast. Embolization was via branches of the right external carotid and the left ophthalmic arteries; left external carotid branches were not accessible because of prior embolization. Early on, when the patient presented with massive epistaxis, embolization was always targeted toward the nasal cavity and nasopharyngeal components of the AVM. Once hemorrhage had largely ceased, different sectors of the AVM were systematically targeted. Embolization with Onyx was staged over seven sessions. Lateral angiographic views of left internal carotid artery injections demonstrating successively less opacification of the AVM following successively more extensive embolization (Q, R, and S, respectively). The ophthalmic artery continues to fill (and there has been no worsening in the already diminished vision in the left eye), but is progressively more difficult to visualize because of the density of the Onyx cast around it. What remains of the AVM is largely nidus supplied directly by angiographically inaccessible cavernous ICA branches (arrow in S).

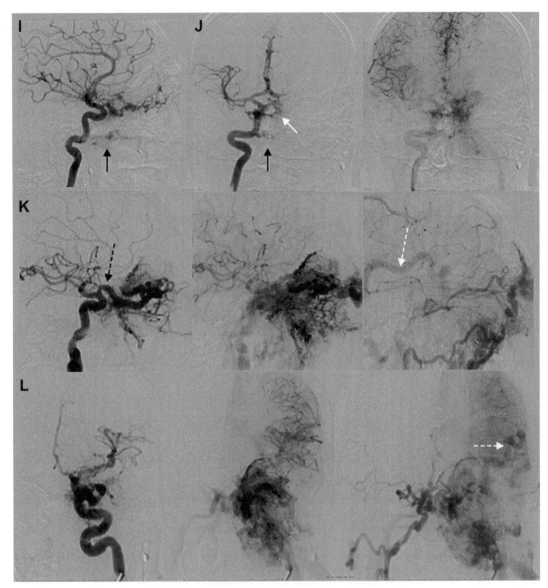

Fig. 3. (*continued*)

nidus is accessible percutaneously, reserving the more invasive and potentially more disfiguring combined embolization/surgery for lesions resistant to sclerotherapy or inaccessible percutaneously.[6] There are also reports of successful cure with embolization alone, but these seemed to be limited to smaller AVMs and long-term follow-up is lacking.[11] The best chance for a complete cure of AVMs of the head and neck seems to be via a combination of preoperative embolization and surgical resection.[5,12,13] If a complete resection is not achievable because of the extent of the lesion or involvement of vital structures, partial targeted endovascular embolization with liquid embolic agents is the treatment of choice.

It is important to emphasize that, regardless of the intended outcomes, proximal embolization of feeding arteries is contraindicated, as is proximal surgical arterial ligation. These not only promote recruitment of nearby arteries to perfuse the nidus (see **Fig. 2**), but also limit future endovascular access to the nidus.[13] By the same token, partial surgical resection of the AVM itself frequently (and perhaps inevitably) leads to progression, and therefore should be reserved only for very

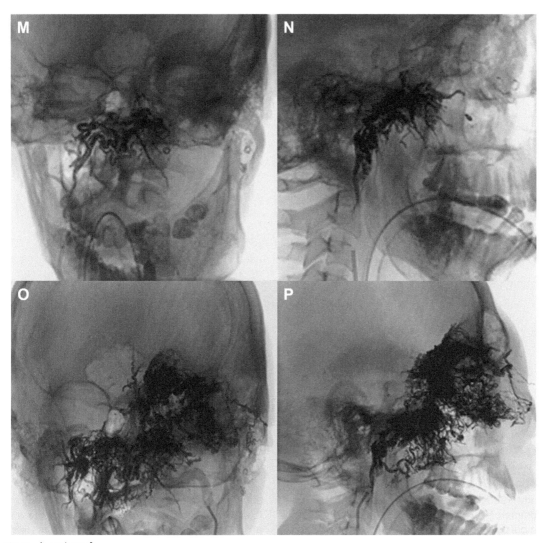

Fig. 3. (*continued*)

rare cases of life-threatening hemorrhage uncontrollable with endovascular or percutaneous embolization.[2,11]

The ultimate target for endovascular embolization is occlusion of the nidus and initial segment of the venous outflow. Embolization may be curative, palliative (for symptomatic control of unresectable lesions), or preoperative, with the choice of agent depending on the intended outcome. For preoperative embolization, temporary occlusive agents such as gelfoam powder, PVA particles, and embospheres can be used. These agents very effectively reduce vascular inflow to AVMs, allowing for significantly lower rates of intraoperative blood loss. PVA and embospheres are available with different particulate diameters, allowing for initial targeting of distal arteriolar branches with small sizes, followed by occlusion of larger, more proximal branches with larger sizes. However, these agents are removed within weeks by phagocytosis, resulting in short-term revascularization. Thus, for embolization that is not to be followed by resection, permanent liquid agents capable of permeating the AVM nidus, such as absolute ethanol, n-BCA, or the more recently available Onyx, may be used.

ENDOVASCULAR EMBOLIZATION WITH ONYX

The use of ethylene-vinyl alcohol copolymer (Onyx, EV3 Neurovascular, Irvine, CA) as an embolic agent for AVMs was first reported in the

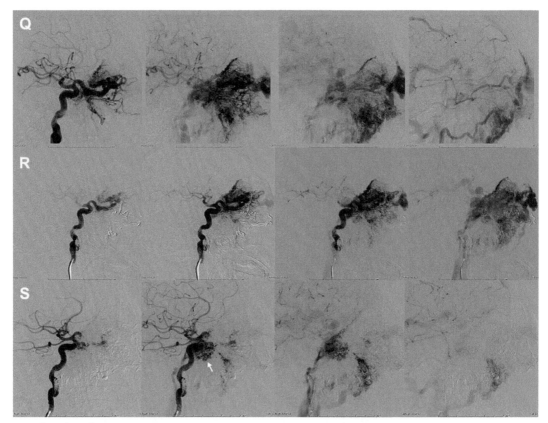

Fig. 3. (*continued*)

early 1990s in Japan.[14,15] It has since become commercially available as a nonadhesive liquid embolic agent under the trade name of Onyx, and is approved by the Food and Drug Administration for use in embolizing brain AVMs.

The availability of Onyx has brought about a sea-change in the embolization of central nervous system AVMs.[16–18] In contact with blood, Onyx precipitates on the surface while maintaining a liquid core, allowing the formation of a nonadhesive lava-like continuous mass. This lowers the risk of fragmentation leading to unintended distal embolization, and offers the user significantly more control with which to aggressively embolize even very extensive AVM nidus and multiple nidal compartments from a single catheter position; this was not feasible with other liquid agents. Its ability to maintain a constant liquid core allows for longer injections and better assessment of the treatment progress. In contrast to agents such as n-BCA or alcohol, Onyx elicits less inflammatory response and causes less endothelial damage and angionecrosis.[19] Vessels embolized with Onyx are filled with a soft, sponge-like

substance and are less fragile than vessels embolized with other agents, perhaps because of less of an inflammatory reaction; these factors likely contribute to its improved handling characteristics during surgical resection.[20]

Despite these advantages in the central nervous system, reports on the use of Onyx for embolizing extracranial AVMs remain scarce.[21] Onyx is black, and concerns have been raised regarding its potential for causing black skin staining for superficial lesions. However, we have found Onyx to be superficially invisible in almost all cases. The potential for skin staining seems to be limited to cases where the AVM has components that are superficial enough to have infiltrated dermal layers. This scenario will inevitably have already led to skin staining and darkening by the AVM itself, rendering any deposited Onyx inconspicuous. At our institution, Onyx has become the embolic agent of choice for treatment of AVMs in the head and neck, allowing us to embolize even the most complex lesions aggressively (**Figs. 3** and **4**). Our experience with its use, both for preoperative and primary embolization, has been very positive.

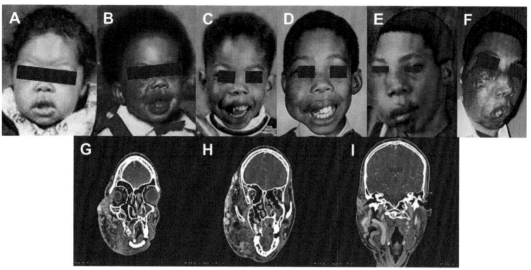

Fig. 4. (*A–F*) Successive growth of a right cheek AVM from infancy through adulthood (ages 2 months, 11 months, 3 years, 8 years, 18 years, and 25 years, respectively). The patient had chronic pain and, at age 22, developed bleeding from points lateral to the right eye and the right upper lip. (*G–I*) Coronal views from a computerized tomographic angiography demonstrate that unlike the case for the patient in Fig. 2, much of the cheek bulk in this case consists of AVM nidus and soft tissue overgrowth. Frontal (*J*) and lateral (*K*) angiographic views of a right external carotid injection demonstrating a diffuse AVM nidus throughout the right temporal fossa, cheek, nose, and supraorbital region. (*L*) Lateral views of a right internal carotid artery injection demonstrate collateral supply to the AVM via mandibular (*black arrow*), cavernous (*white arrow*) and ophthalmic branches. Frontal (*M*) and lateral (*N*) unsubtracted fluoroscopic views demonstrating the Onyx cast after staged embolization. Frontal (*O*) and lateral (*P*) angiographic views of a right external carotid injection after embolization demonstrating reduced flow to the AVM, with minimal early venous opacification. The patient is asymptomatic and awaiting targeted resection.

HIGH-FLOW VASCULAR MALFORMATIONS AT SPECIFIC SITES IN THE HEAD AND NECK

As mentioned previously, HFVMs of the head and neck favor several primary sites, occurring most commonly in the cheek (31%), followed by the ear (16%) and nose (11%).[5] Anatomic and functional challenges posed by particular locations in the head and neck impart a level of complexity to the management of these AVMs that is often lacking at other sites in the body. Here we consider several head and neck sites where HFVMs present unique treatment challenges.

Ear

The ear is the second most common site for AVMs of the head and neck. In the largest series of auricular AVMs, approximately 66% of the cases were noted at birth as a "vascular birthmark" of the ear, with the balance either absent or clinically not apparent.[22] As expected, the most common feeding arteries were the posterior auricular, superficial temporal, and occipital arteries (see Fig. 2).

Signs and symptoms depend upon the clinical stage of the lesion. The most common signs are macrotia, erythema, bleeding, pain, bruit, or thrill. We are not aware of any reports of auricular AVM having progressed to stage IV. Similar to AVMs in other sites of the head and neck, most patients note enlargement of the lesions in response to hormonal changes (eg, puberty or, pregnancy) or trauma. While extra-auricular involvement is seen in over 90% of the cases (most commonly in the retroauricular or cheek/parotid regions), the middle and inner ear structures are virtually never involved.[22] Because a stage I lesion may remain stable for a lengthy period of time, our practice is to recommend conservative management for stage I and II lesions, with intervention considered only with the onset of significant symptomatology.[22]

The definitive treatment for auricular AVMs remains surgical resection (ie, total or partial amputation), preferably with preoperative embolization, which provides a dry surgical field and minimizes perioperative blood loss. Interestingly, however,

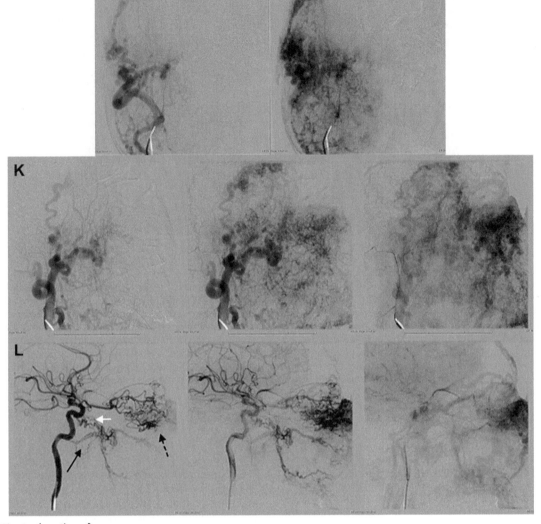

Fig. 4. (*continued*)

the margin of resection is not altered with preoperative embolization.[7,22–24] Given that much of the arterial supply to auricular AVMs involves end-arteries, therapeutic embolization in this location is particularly fraught with risk. Nevertheless, some authors have reported success with selective embolization, even using ethanol, in this location.[25] Attempts at total angiographic cure are likely to lead to tissue ischemia necessitating amputation; on the other hand, more limited, targeted embolization may offer an improvement in symptoms that may last up to several years.[22,26,27] Therefore, although ultimately most auricular AMV patients are likely to face amputation, selective palliative embolization is an important part of the therapeutic armamentarium.

Mandible and Maxilla

The mandible and maxilla are uncommon sites for HFVMs of the head and neck, accounting for less than 10% of the cases.[5] Trauma or surgery may result in a pure AVF in this location, but the overwhelming majority of congenital cases are AVMs.[12,28,29] AVMs in the maxilla or mandible can pose a risk of life-threatening hemorrhage associated with dental procedures or tooth eruption.[30,31]

AVM of the maxilla is characteristically supplied by the distal branches of the internal maxillary artery, with frequent contribution from branches of the ascending pharyngeal artery and the superior labial branch of the facial

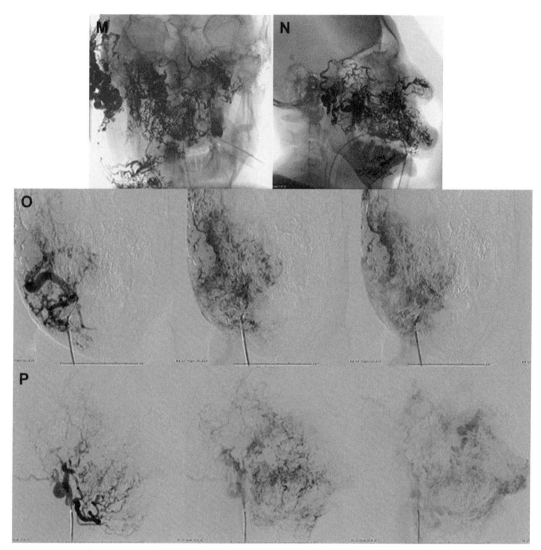

Fig. 4. (*continued*)

artery; posterior ethmoidal branches of the ophthalmic artery are frequently recruited as well.[11] Mandibular AVMs are most commonly supplied by the inferior alveolar branch of the internal maxillary, as well as by branches of the facial and lingual arteries.

Surgical management of these lesions is particularly challenging because of the skeletal involvement. It is interesting to note that primary bony involvement of AVMs of the head and neck occurs only in the tooth-bearing bones such as mandible and maxilla. Resection for cure in these cases involves a bony excision. In contradistinction, secondary bony involvement (ie, osseous erosion by adjacent soft tissue AVMs or indentation by enlarged draining veins)

does not necessitate excision of bony structures for potential cure.[5]

Although endovascular embolization alone as the definitive treatment has been reported,[32] most series report only temporary relief, and many authors recommend a combined regimen.[2,31,33] Some authors advocate endovascular embolization with direct injection of adhesive into the bony nidus and draining veins, which may result in complete nidal ablation with reossification of the affected mandible.[11,34] Others advocate endovascular embolization followed by tooth extraction or surgical excision. However, the total cure rate is significantly lower than AVMs in other regions of the head and neck, and we have seen AVM recurrence after aggressive embolization

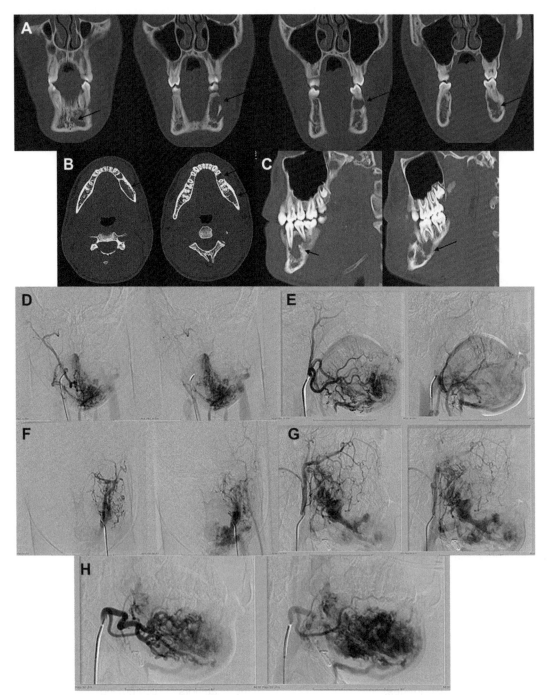

Fig. 5. Coronal (*A*), axial (*B*), and sagittal (*C*) views of a high-resolution computerized tomographic angiography demonstrating osseous lucencies indicative of bony involvement by a mandibular and floor of mouth AVM. The 16-year-old patient had mild loosening of some left lower teeth, intermittent bloody spotting of his toothbrush, and occasional aching in the lower lateral left jaw. Right external carotid angiogram, in frontal (*D*) and lateral (*E*) views. Left ECA injection, in frontal (*F*) and lateral (*G*) views. (*H*) Lateral view of a selective left facial artery injection. Venous collectors are visible as intramandibular fluffy foci of opacification (see overlap with the Onyx cast in (*I*). (*I*) Frontal and lateral unsubtracted fluoroscopic views demonstrating the Onyx cast filling the venous lakes in the left mandible. Successive views of a right (*J*) and left (*K*) external carotid artery injection, in lateral view. There is minimal residual abnormal opacification, with no significant arteriovenous shunting. Increased flow to the right lower lip may portend future AVM growth at that site, but this area has been asymptomatic thus far.

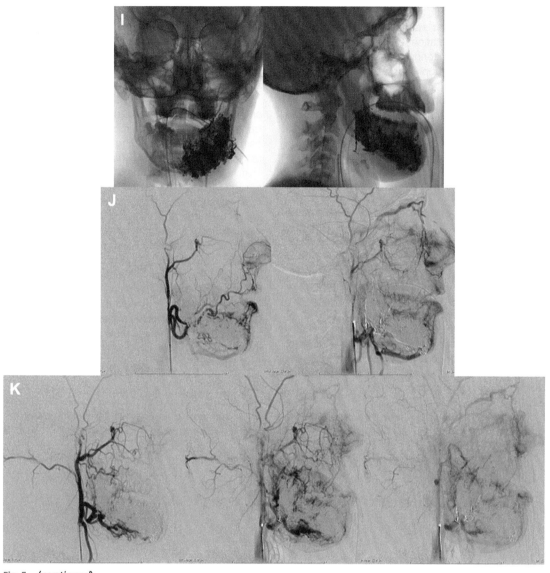

Fig. 5. (continued)

and disfiguring maxillectomy. Therefore, our main treatment goal for extensive AVMs in these regions is long-term symptom control rather than attempted total lesion eradication.[5,11] Although we typically embolize transarterially, to ensure lasting results, the ultimate targets are the intraosseous draining venous lakes (Fig. 5).

One reported drawback to using acrylic embolization agents for maxillary and mandibular AVMs is the development of foreign body reaction, leading to sequestered bone or infection, potentially requiring subsequent debridement. Infected n-BCA has been reported to extrude from sockets after the loss of teeth.[2] Early studies suggest that

Onyx incites less angionecrosis and endothelial denudation,[35,36] which at least theoretically may represent an advantage for peridental AVMs. We have not encountered foreign body reaction or Onyx extrusion after embolization of lesions in these locations, but long-term follow-up is still pending.

Tongue

The tongue is a rare location for AVMs, and most cases are diffuse AVMs with tongue and floor of mouth involvement.[37–39] Left untreated, these lesions can grow significantly, with macroglossia causing both cosmetic and functional interference. Despite the inherent vascularity of the tongue, aggressive embolization can lead to tissue ischemia and even tongue loss entirely (Fig. 6). The main arterial supply for AVM of the tongue region is the lingual artery, with supplemental supply from the submental branch of facial artery or the sublingual branches of the superior thyroidal artery.[37,38] Targeted embolization and even partial glossectomy may be necessary to maintain speech and swallowing viability.[37]

Scalp

The scalp is another rare location for HFVMs of the head and neck, with fewer than 60 cases reported in the literature.[40] As noted earlier, at all other locations, AVM is far more common than AVF. However, in the scalp, most HFVMs are AVFs. The characteristic variceal dilatation of the draining veins are referred to as the cirsoid aneurysm of the scalp (from the Greek kirsos, or varix).[40,41] While there are reports of siblings with homologous occipital cirsoid aneurysms present at birth, suggesting a congenital origin,[42] many cases occur after head trauma, such as craniotomy, hair transplantation, or intravenous infusion via scalp veins.[41]

Regardless of etiology, similar to other HFVMs of the head and neck, scalp AVFs typically begin as a small, subcutaneous, discolored lump in the scalp, progressing over time into a large deforming mass. In the vast majority of cases, the main arterial supply is the superficial temporal artery, with frequent involvement of the posterior auricular and occipital arteries as well.[41,43]

Traditionally, surgical resection of the cirsoid aneurysm was considered to be the most effective treatment.[40,41,44] However, particularly in fistulous cases with a single feeding artery, endovascular techniques can be highly effective, both for preoperative adjunctive treatment and as a stand-alone cure (Fig. 7).[43] In cases where multiple small feeders supply a nidus, nidal embolization followed by surgical resection is the usual treatment prescription. Occasionally a wide swath of scalp is involved, necessitating a large resection. The use of tissue expanders has been advocated by some in this context,[45,46] although others prefer resection followed by skin grafts or tissue flaps.[40,41,47] There is at least the theoretical possibility that the use of tissue expanders in this setting may serve as an angiogenesis promoter, resulting in AVM proliferation, although this has never been documented.

Orbit and Nose

The orbits are rare sites for HFVMs of the head and neck, and the true incidence at this site is

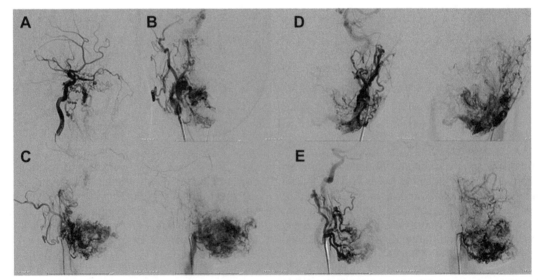

Fig. 6. Lateral view of a right internal carotid (A), frontal (B), and lateral (C) views of a right external carotid, and frontal (D) and lateral (E) views of a left external carotid injection. The patient had an AVM of the tongue and floor of mouth that involved the mandible. She is status post mandibulectomy and lost her tongue entirely to necrosis after prior alcohol embolization (but is able, remarkably, to speak clearly, and has no dysphagia). She presents with recurrent AVM causing oral pain. As we have seen previously, the AVM has recruited mandibular, cavernous, and ophthalmic ICA supply, as well as bilateral ECA supply.

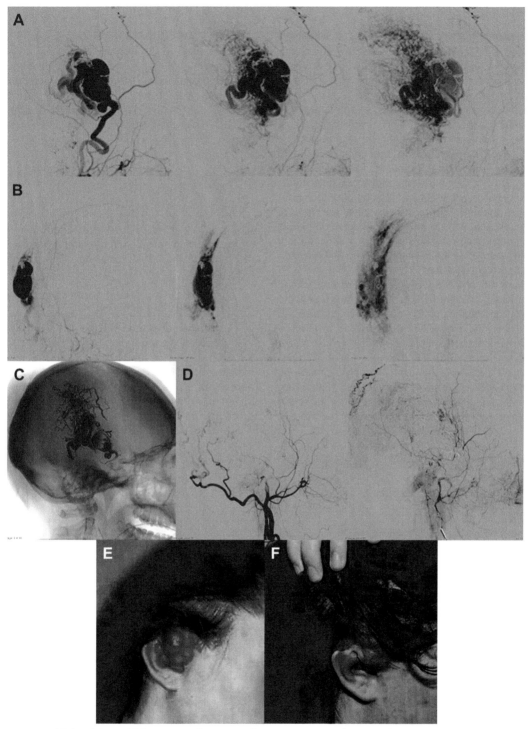

Fig. 7. Lateral (*A*) and frontal (*B*) angiographic views of successive images from a right external carotid artery injection. The patient was transferred from another hospital with massive scalp bleeding that was difficult to control, requiring multiple transfusions. There had been prior embolizations with coils and alcohol. The superficial temporal artery is aneurysmally dilated at the point of its communication with the AVM nidus; there was no clear fistula. On the frontal views, note the overgrowth of scalp thickness and the extent of involvement by AVM. Lateral unsubtracted fluoroscopic view of the Onyx cast (*C*), approximating the morphology of the feeding artery aneurysm and nidus seen in *A*. Serial lateral angiographic images (*D*) from a right external carotid injection following embolization, demonstrating no significant residual AVM opacification. Photograph taken soon before the most severe episode of massive bleeding occurred (*E*), and comparison photograph taken after staged embolization (*F*). Note the decrement in size of the auricular soft tissue mass and its less intensely red color.

unknown.[48] Orbital AVMs have been described, based upon their predominant location, as anterior (involving or adjacent to the lids, or preseptal) or posterior (intraconal, or postseptal). These malformations may present with primary orbital signs, such as proptosis or chemosis, and/or symptoms related to optic nerve dysfunction and orbital venous congestion. The major arterial supply for orbital AVMs may involve branches of external carotid artery, the ophthalmic artery, or both (Fig. 8).[48–50] These lesions post a particular treatment challenge because of the complex neurovascular anatomy in the region and the risk of hemorrhage, with its attendant neuro-ophthalmic complications.[51] Not surprisingly, many authors favor a combined treatment involving embolization and surgical excision.[51–53]

Pure retinal AVMs are rare, but there is increased incidence in Wyburn Mason syndrome (see the following section). Unlike other AVMs of the head and neck, these retinal AVMs usually do no undergo rapid progression, but rather typically remain stable and asymptomatic without any treatment.[54] Therefore, retinal AVMs may require only surveillance rather than aggressive intervention.[54] However, a rare case of glaucoma related to retinal ischemia from arteriovenous shunting has been reported.[55]

Nasal AVMs usually have collateral supply via the ophthalmic artery. Unless there has already been diminution of normal visual function, embolization is performed via the external carotid supply, so as not to subject ipsilateral vision to undue risk. Patients almost always present with epistaxis, which can be severe, requiring chronic transfusion (Fig. 9).

SYNDROMES ASSOCIATED WITH ARTERIOVENOUS MALFORMATIONS OF THE HEAD AND NECK

Although rare, HFVMs of the head and neck are associated with several nonhereditary and hereditary conditions. The following are selected examples.

Nonhereditary Conditions

It has been demonstrated that the neural crest and the adjacent mesodermal cells originate from a shared transverse level in the cephalic region (a metamere).[56] Thus, disorders affecting the development of these cells before their subsequent migration may produce malformations with a segmental distribution. These have been

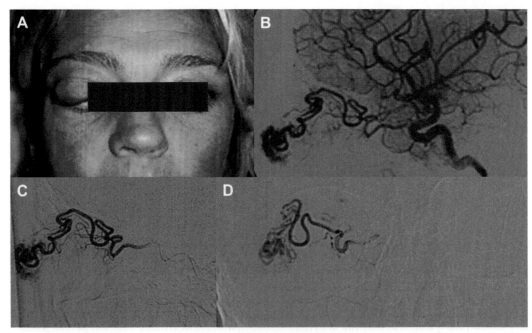

Fig. 8. (A) Right orbital AVM. The patient's right eyelid had always been more prominent than the left, but underwent dramatic growth during both the patient's pregnancies. Progressive pro ptosis precluded normal binocular vision. Lateral right internal carotid (B) and lateral (C) and frontal (D) selective right ophthalmic artery injections demonstrate that the arterial supply is entirely via a single enlarged supraorbital branch of the ophthalmic artery, and the nidus is entirely confined to the lid, making this a preseptal AVM. Hemostasis was readily obtained under direct observation during surgery, and preoperative embolization was not necessary.

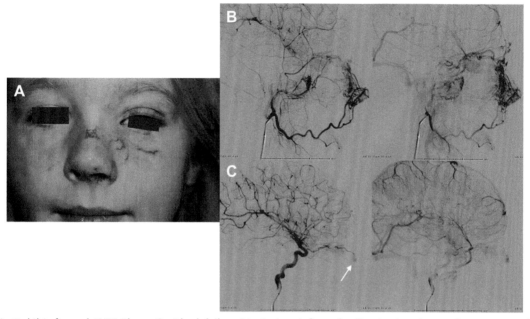

Fig. 9. (A) Left nasal AVM. The patient had daily epistaxis since infancy, leading to chronic anemia, most recently requiring transfusions. Diagnosis of AVM was delayed until age 5. Lateral left external carotid (B) and internal carotid (C) injections demonstrating the main arterial supply to the AVM to be the left internal maxillary artery. The left ophthalmic artery supplied a component of the AVM in the eyelid (arrow); this was asymptomatic. (D) Unsubtracted fluoroscopic views demonstrating the Onyx cast. (E) Lateral views of the left external carotid injection after embolization, demonstrate nonopacification of the nasal component of the AVM. The eyelid component is still visible (arrow). The epistaxis has resolved and the patient is no longer anemic.

collectively referred to as the cerebrofacial arteriovenous metameric syndromes.[57]

To take a particular example, Wyburn Mason syndrome (or Bonnet-Dechaume-Blanc syndrome) is a rare condition characterized by paired head and neck and intracranial AVMs. There are frequently associated retinal vascular malformations, typically ipsilateral to the brain lesion. The facial AVMs are generally Schobinger stage I lesions, which may demonstrate unilateral involvement of the skin in the trigeminal nerve distribution, or a more central involvement of the mid forehead, glabella, nose, and upper lip.[58,59] Rare bilateral cases have been reported.[60] The retinal and facial AVMs are typically stable, and most patients are managed conservatively with observation. There is no evidence that cerebral AVMs in Wyburn Mason syndrome behave differently from isolated cerebral AVMs, and thus management is similar to that of cerebral AVMs not associated with Wyburn Mason.[59]

Hereditary Arteriovenous Malformations of the Head and Neck

The vast majority of AVMs are sporadic, and they have been generally considered nonhereditary in

the past; however, recent studies have identified syndromes involving head and neck HFVMs with corresponding genetic markers. For example, gene mutations involving endoglin and ALK-1, binding proteins for transforming growth factor (TGF)-beta, result in defective development of the endothelial cell layer in AVMs and are associated with Osler-Weber-Rendu syndrome.[61] Similarly in the head and neck, AVMs have been observed in conditions such as capillary malformation-AVM syndrome (CM-AVM) and posphatase and tensin (PTEN) homologue mutation.

CM-AVM syndrome is a hereditary disorder characterized by cutaneous capillary malformations (CMs) with associated HFVMs.[62] This disorder is caused by mutations in the RASA-1 gene, which encodes a protein critical in the signaling pathway for proliferation, migration, and survival of endothelial cells. Variable phenotypes have been observed, and HFVMs can occur in the head and neck as cutaneous, subcutaneous, intramuscular, or intraosseous AVMs or AVFs. Intracranial HFVMs can also occur.[62,63]

Another mutation associated with AVMs of the head and neck involves the PTEN gene, which encodes a tumor suppressor protein that regulates

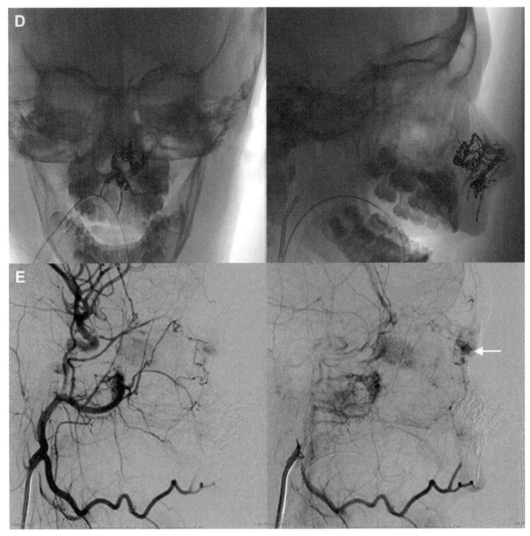

Fig. 9. (continued)

the pathway involving cell-cycle regulation, angiogenesis, and cellular growth and proliferation. PTEN mutations occur in syndromes that have been known by a variety of eponyms, such as Cowden syndrome and Bannayan-Riley-Ruvalcaba syndrome (BRRS).[64] Among the patients with PTEN mutations (now designated as PTEN hamartoma-tumor syndrome or PHTS), more than half (54%) have vascular anomalies.[65] Radiographically, these vascular anomalies of the head and neck are all consistent with high-flow lesions, with at least some degree of AV shunting (Fig. 10). However, there are histological and radiographical features that differentiate these high-flow lesions from typical AVMs. Ectopic

fat within or adjacent to the lesion, with disruption of the architecture of the affected muscle, is common, as is disproportionate dilation of the draining veins. In addition, involvement of multiple noncontiguous sites is commonly seen with PHTS patients, and is rare in patients with nonsyndromic AVM. Other clinical manifestations of PHTS include prominence of the brow, macrocrania, and penile freckling.[65]

At our institution, the patients who present with multiple high-flow vascular anomalies or anomalies with the features mentioned previously are carefully screened for other clinical features of PHTS, and molecular PTEN testing is considered. Given the associated risk of various benign and

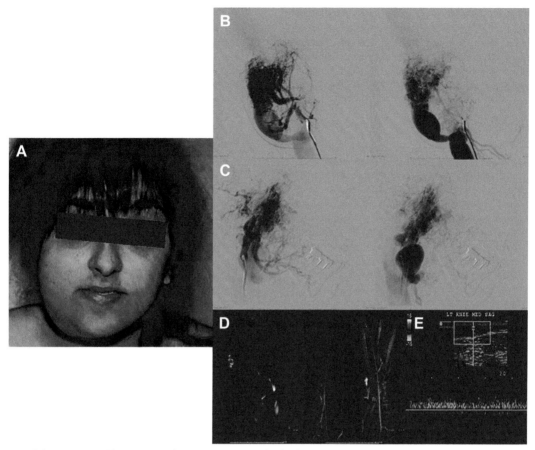

Fig. 10. (A) A 21-year-old woman with PTEN mutation. She had a right cheek and temporal fossa mass that grew steadily through her teenage years. Other than effect on cosmesis, she has been entirely asymptomatic. She underwent prior embolization and resection of the temporal fossa component at an outside institution, with placement of a tissue expander. Frontal (B) and lateral (C) views of a right external carotid injection demonstrate a diffuse nidus in the right temporal fossa and cheek, with ectatic venous drainage creating much of the bulk of the visible mass (similar to the case in Fig. 2). It is difficult to outline discrete feeding arteries; rather, the superficial temporal artery seems to give rise diffusely to nidal vessels. During the course of staged embolization, the patient complained of left knee pain and swelling, and was found on MR (D) and sonographic examination (E) to have a small knee AVM as well.

malignant tumors, the diagnosis of PTEN mutation is important, as it triggers appropriate multisystem surveillance.

SUMMARY

Head and neck high-flow vascular malformations are uncommon lesions whose management presents a clinical challenge. Although in some rare cases a complete cure is possible, in the vast majority the primary objective is symptom control, cosmesis improvement, and preservation of vital functions. Striving for "complete cure" in most cases results in potentially devastating clinical and cosmetic outcome. Collateral supply via intra-cranial vessels is not uncommon, and scrupulous efforts to avoid complications related to inadvertent intracranial embolization or venous thrombosis are mandatory. Regardless of the therapeutic goal, close long-term follow-up for recurrence of the lesions is necessary. Recent demonstration of syndromic associations for some subsets of HFVMs holds out the promise of the future development of medical therapy for these difficult lesions.

ACKNOWLEDGMENTS

The authors express their profound indebtedness to the physicians and staff of the Vascular Anomalies Center at Children's Hospital Boston, headed by Drs. John B. Mulliken and Stephen J. Fishman, and to Dr. Patricia E. Burrows, who was involved with earlier treatment of several of the patients discussed here. Additionally, the authors thank the staff of the Interventional Radiology Division at Children's Hospital Boston and the Neurointerventional Service at Brigham and Women's Hospital.

REFERENCES

1. Mulliken JB, Glowacki J. Hemangiomas and vascular malformations in infants and children: a classification based on endothelial characteristics. Plast Reconstr Surg 1982;69:412–22.
2. Niimi Y, Song JK, Berenstein A. Current endovascular management of maxillofacial vascular malformations. Neuroimaging Clin N Am 2007;17:223–37.
3. Garzon MC, Huang JT, Enjolras O, et al. Vascular malformations: part I. J Am Acad Dermatol 2007; 56:353–70 [quiz 371–354].
4. Van Aalst JA, Bhuller A, Sadove AM. Pediatric vascular lesions. J Craniofac Surg 2003;14:566–83.
5. Kohout MP, Hansen M, Pribaz JJ, et al. Arteriovenous malformations of the head and neck: natural history and management. Plast Reconstr Surg 1998;102:643–54.
6. Jeong HS, Baek CH, Son YI, et al. Treatment for extracranial arteriovenous malformations of the head and neck. Acta Otolaryngol 2006;126: 295–300.
7. Bradley JP, Zide BM, Berenstein A, et al. Large arteriovenous malformations of the face: aesthetic results with recurrence control. Plast Reconstr Surg 1999;103:351–61.
8. Ziyeh S, Schumacher M, Strecker R, et al. Head and neck vascular malformations: time-resolved MR projection angiography. Neuroradiology 2003;45: 681–6.
9. Ziyeh S, Strecker R, Berlis A, et al. Dynamic 3D MR angiography of intra- and extracranial vascular malformations at 3T: a technical note. AJNR Am J Neuroradiol 2005;26:630–4.
10. Paltiel HJ, Burrows PE, Kozakewich HP, et al. Soft-tissue vascular anomalies: utility of US for diagnosis. Radiology 2000;214:747–54.
11. Persky MS, Yoo HJ, Berenstein A. Management of vascular malformations of the mandible and maxilla. Laryngoscope 2003;113:1885–92.
12. Kim BS, Lee SK, terBrugge KG. Endovascular treatment of congenital arteriovenous fistulae of the internal maxillary artery. Neuroradiology 2003;45: 445–50.
13. Turowski B, Zanella FE. Interventional neuroradiology of the head and neck. Neuroimaging Clin N Am 2003;13:619–45.
14. Taki W, Yonekawa Y, Iwata H, et al. A new liquid material for embolization of arteriovenous malformations. AJNR Am J Neuroradiol 1990;11:163–8.
15. Terada T, Nakamura Y, Nakai K, et al. Embolization of arteriovenous malformations with peripheral aneurysms using ethylene vinyl alcohol copolymer. Report of three cases. J Neurosurg 1991;75: 655–60.
16. Jahan R, Murayama Y, Gobin YP, et al. Embolization of arteriovenous malformations with Onyx: clinico-pathological experience in 23 patients. Neurosurgery 2001;48:984–95 [discussion: 995–7].
17. Mounayer C, Hammami N, Piotin M, et al. Nidal embolization of brain arteriovenous malformations using Onyx in 94 patients. AJNR Am J Neuroradiol 2007;28:518–23.
18. van Rooij WJ, Sluzewski M, Beute GN. Brain AVM embolization with Onyx. AJNR Am J Neuroradiol 2007;28:172–7 [discussion: 178].
19. Duffner F, Ritz R, Bornemann A, et al. Combined therapy of cerebral arteriovenous malformations: histological differences between a non-adhesive liquid embolic agent and n-butyl 2-cyanoacrylate (NBCA). Clin Neuropathol 2002;21:13–7.
20. Akin ED, Perkins E, Ross IB. Surgical handling characteristics of an ethylene vinyl alcohol copolymer compared with N-butyl cyanoacrylate used for embolization of vessels in an arteriovenous malformation resection model in swine. J Neurosurg 2003;98:366–70.
21. Arat A, Cil BE, Vargel I, et al. Embolization of high-flow craniofacial vascular malformations with Onyx. AJNR Am J Neuroradiol 2007;28:1409–14.
22. Wu JK, Bisdorff A, Gelbert F, et al. Auricular arteriovenous malformation: evaluation, management, and outcome. Plast Reconstr Surg 2005;115:985–95.
23. Pham TH, Wong BJ, Allison G. A large arteriovenous malformation of the external ear in an adult: report of a case and approach to management. Laryngoscope 2001;111:1390–4.
24. Meher R, Varshney S, Pant HC. Arteriovenous malformation related to the pinna. Hong Kong Med J 2008;14:157–9.
25. Yakes WF, Rossi P, Odink H. How I do it. Arteriovenous malformation management. Cardiovasc Intervent Radiol 1996;19:65–71.
26. Shinohara K, Yamashita M, Sugimoto K, et al. Transcatheter arterial embolization of auricular arteriovenous malformation. Otolaryngol Head Neck Surg 2005;132:345–6.
27. Erdmann MW, Jackson JE, Davies DM, et al. Multidisciplinary approach to the management of head and neck arteriovenous malformations. Ann R Coll Surg Engl 1995;77:53–9.
28. Halbach VV, Higashida RT, Hieshima GB, et al. Arteriovenous fistula of the internal maxillary artery: treatment with transarterial embolization. Radiology 1988;168:443–5.
29. Saini A, Jackson JE. Arteriovenous fistulas of the facial artery after mandibular surgery: treatment by

embolization. AJR Am J Roentgenol 2008;190: W35–40.

30. Engel JD, Supancic JS, Davis LF. Arteriovenous malformation of the mandible: life-threatening complications during tooth extraction. J Am Dent Assoc 1995; 126:237–42.

31. Sakkas N, Schramm A, Metzger MC, et al. Arteriovenous malformation of the mandible: a life-threatening situation. Ann Hematol 2007;86:409–13.

32. Kiyosue H, Mori H, Hori Y, et al. Treatment of mandibular arteriovenous malformation by transvenous embolization: a case report. Head Neck 1999;21:574–7.

33. Jackson IT, Jack CR, Aycock B, et al. The management of intraosseous arteriovenous malformations in the head and neck area. Plast Reconstr Surg 1989; 84:47–54.

34. Corsten L, Bashir Q, Thornton J, et al. Treatment of a giant mandibular arteriovenous malformation with percutaneous embolization using histoacrylic glue: a case report. J Oral Maxillofac Surg 2001;59: 828–32.

35. Gobin YP, Murayama Y, Milanese K, et al. Head and neck hypervascular lesions: embolization with ethylene vinyl alcohol copolymer—laboratory evaluation in swine and clinical evaluation in humans. Radiology 2001;221:309–17.

36. Mazal PR, Stichenwirth M, Gruber A, et al. Tissue reactions induced by different embolising agents in cerebral arteriovenous malformations: a histopathological follow-up. Pathology 2006;38: 28–32.

37. Richter GT, Suen J, North PE, et al. Arteriovenous malformations of the tongue: a spectrum of disease. Laryngoscope 2007;117:328–35.

38. Slaba S, Herbreteau D, Jhaveri HS, et al. Therapeutic approach to arteriovenous malformations of the tongue. Eur Radiol 1998;8:280–5.

39. Righi PD, Bade MA, Coleman JJ 3rd, et al. Arteriovenous malformation of the base of tongue: case report and literature review. Microsurgery 1996;17: 706–9.

40. Gurkanlar D, Gonul M, Solmaz I, et al. Cirsoid aneurysms of the scalp. Neurosurg Rev 2006;29:208–12.

41. Muthukumar N, Rajagopal V, Manoharan AV, et al. Surgical management of cirsoid aneurysms. Acta Neurochir (Wien) 2002;144:349–56.

42. Khodadad G. Familial cirsoid aneurysm of the scalp. J Neurol Neurosurg Psychiatry 1971;34:664–7.

43. Barnwell SL, Halbach VV, Dowd CF, et al. Endovascular treatment of scalp arteriovenous fistulas associated with a large varix. Radiology 1989;173: 533–9.

44. Corr PD. Cirsoid aneurysm of the scalp. Singapore Med J 2007;48:e268–9.

45. Marotta TR, Berenstein A, Zide B. The combined role of embolization and tissue expanders in the management of arteriovenous malformations of the scalp. AJNR Am J Neuroradiol 1994;15: 1240–6.

46. Nagasaka S, Fukushima T, Goto K, et al. Treatment of scalp arteriovenous malformation. Neurosurgery 1996;38:671–7 [discussion: 677].

47. Tiwary SK, Khanna R, Khanna AK. Craniofacial cirsoid aneurysm: 2-stage treatment. J Oral Maxillofac Surg 2007;65:523–5.

48. Huna-Baron R, Setton A, Kupersmith MJ, et al. Orbital arteriovenous malformation mimicking cavernous sinus dural arteriovenous malformation. Br J Ophthalmol 2000;84:771–4.

49. Moin M, Kersten RC, Bernardini F, et al. Spontaneous hemorrhage in an intraorbital arteriovenous malformation. Ophthalmology 2000;107: 2215–9.

50. Gil-Salu JL, Gonzalez-Darder JM, Vera-Roman JM. Intraorbital arteriovenous malformation: case report. Skull Base 2004;14:31–6 [discussion: 36–37].

51. Trombly R, Sandberg DI, Wolfe SA, et al. High-flow orbital arteriovenous malformation in a child: current management and options. J Craniofac Surg 2006; 17:779–82.

52. Goldberg RA, Garcia GH, Duckwiler GR. Combined embolization and surgical treatment of arteriovenous malformation of the orbit. Am J Ophthalmol 1993; 116:17–25.

53. Hayes BH, Shore JW, Westfall CT, et al. Management of orbital and periorbital arteriovenous malformations. Ophthalmic Surg 1995;26:145–52.

54. Reck SD, Zacks DN, Eibschitz-Tsimhoni M. Retinal and intracranial arteriovenous malformations: Wyburn-Mason syndrome. J Neuroophthalmol 2005;25:205–8.

55. Effron L, Zakov ZN, Tomsak RL. Neovascular glaucoma as a complication of the Wyburn-Mason syndrome. J Clin Neuroophthalmol 1985; 5:95–8.

56. Couly G, Coltey P, Eichmann A, et al. The angiogenic potentials of the cephalic mesoderm and the origin of brain and head blood vessels. Mech Dev 1995;53:97–112.

57. Krings T, Geibprasert S, Luo CB, et al. Segmental neurovascular syndromes in children. Neuroimaging Clin N Am 2007;17:245–58.

58. Brodsky MC, Hoyt WF. Spontaneous involution of retinal and intracranial arteriovenous malformation in Bonnet-Dechaume-Blanc syndrome. Br J Ophthalmol 2002;86:360–1.

59. Dayani PN, Sadun AA. A case report of Wyburn-Mason syndrome and review of the literature. Neuroradiology 2007;49:445–56.

60. Kim J, Kim OH, Suh JH, et al. Wyburn-Mason syndrome: an unusual presentation of bilateral orbital and unilateral brain arteriovenous malformations. Pediatr Radiol 1998;28:161.

61. Tille JC, Pepper MS. Hereditary vascular anomalies: new insights into their pathogenesis. Arterioscler Thromb Vasc Biol 2004;24:1578–90.

62. Boon LM, Mulliken JB, Vikkula M. RASA1: variable phenotype with capillary and arteriovenous malformations. Curr Opin Genet Dev 2005;15:265–9.

63. Eerola I, Boon LM, Mulliken JB, et al. Capillary malformation—arteriovenous malformation, a new clinical and genetic disorder caused by RASA1 mutations. Am J Hum Genet 2003;73:1240–9.

64. Eng C. PTEN: one gene, many syndromes. Hum Mutat 2003;22:183–98.

65. Tan WH, Baris HN, Burrows PE, et al. The spectrum of vascular anomalies in patients with PTEN mutations: implications for diagnosis and management. J Med Genet 2007;44:594–602.

Endovascular Treatment of Carotid Cavernous Fistulas

Joseph J. Gemmete, MD[a,*], Sameer A. Ansari, MD, PhD[a],
Dheeraj Gandhi, MD[b,c]

KEYWORDS

- Carotid cavernous fistula • Endovascular treatment
- Classification • Etiology and pathology
- Clinical presentation

This article provides an overview of direct and indirect carotid cavernous fistulas (CCFs) with emphasis on the recent advances in endovascular techniques available for treatment. It first briefly discusses the classification, etiology and pathology, clinical presentation, and diagnostic imaging of direct and indirect CCFs. Additionally, it provides a brief description of the medical management and surgical treatment of direct and indirect CCFs. The subsequent sections present a detailed discussion of the various endovascular techniques available for the treatment of direct and indirect CCFs with a brief discussion of the complications and results of treatment.

CLASSIFICATION

CCFs can be classified based on etiology (traumatic or spontaneous), rate of flow (high versus low flow), or the angiographic architecture (direct or indirect). The most commonly used classification scheme established by Barrow and colleagues[1] divides the CCFs into four types, depending on the arterial supply. Direct (type A fistulas) are direct communications between the internal carotid artery (ICA) and the cavernous sinus, usually associated with high flow rates. Indirect fistulas (types B, C, and D) are dural arteriovenous fistulas (DAVFs) fed by the meningeal arteries of the ICA, the external carotid artery (ECA), or

both. Type B fistulas are relatively uncommon and are supplied only by the dural branches of the ICA. Type C fistulas are supplied solely by the dural branches of the ECA. The most common indirect CCF is a type D fistula, which is supplied by the meningeal branches of both the ICA and ECA.

ETIOLOGY AND PATHOLOGY

Direct (type A) fistulas usually are traumatic, caused by motor vehicle accidents or penetrating injuries,[2] and generally affect young males. Approximately 20% of type A CCFs may be spontaneous, resulting from the rupture of either a cavernous ICA aneurysm or a weakened ICA vessel wall coursing through the cavernous sinus.[3]

Debrun[4] described the site of CCF origin by dividing the cavernous ICA into five arbitrary segments. He found the most common site of occurrence is the proximal horizontal portion of the ICA near the artery of the inferior cavernous sinus (40%). CCFs occur with decreasing frequency at the junction of the horizontal and posterior vertical ascending cavernous segment (28%), at the origins from the posterior vertical ascending segment itself (20%), and distally near the anterior genu and the clinoidal segment (12%).

Van Dellen[5] considers CCFs to be part of a continuum of injury to the arterial and venous

[a] Division of Interventional Neuroradiology, Department of Radiology, University of Michigan Health System, 1500 E. Medical Center Dr., B1D330, Ann Arbor, MI 48109 0030, USA
[b] Department of Radiology, Johns Hopkins Hospital, Baltimore, MD, USA
[c] Department of Neurosurgery, Johns Hopkins Hospital, Baltimore, MD, USA
* Corresponding author.
E-mail address: gemmete@umich.edu (J.J. Gemmete).

Neuroimag Clin N Am 19 (2009) 241–255
doi:10.1016/j.nic.2009.01.006
1052-5149/09/$ – see front matter © 2009 Elsevier Inc. All rights reserved.

vessel wall. An incomplete tear can result in a pseudoaneurysm of the cavernous carotid artery that can compress the venous sinusoids. A true CCF, however, occurs when the arterial tear is complete and there is associated breach of the walls of venous sinusoids.

Flow rates in type A fistulas are variable and depend on the size of the ostium and venous drainage. Complete steal of ICA flow to CCF occurs in approximately 5% of cases at diagnosis. Most fistula ostia measure 2.6 mm in diameter,[4] typically small enough to be treated with detachable balloons with a mean volume of 0.28 cm^3, equivalent to an inflated balloon dimension of 7 mm × 9 mm. Bilateral CCFs occur in approximately 1% to 2% of patients who have traumatic CCFs.[6,7]

Spontaneous direct (type A) CCFs are more common in older women, although a few have been reported in children.[8,9] They usually are caused by the rupture of a cavernous aneurysm or by the spontaneous rupture of a congenitally weakened, atherosclerotic, or diseased artery. Predisposition to spontaneous direct CCFs have been shown in fibromuscular dysplasia, Ehlers-Danlos syndrome, and pseudoxanthoma elasticum.[10,11]

Indirect (types B, C, or D) CCFs have a predilection for spontaneous occurrence in postmenopausal women. Sinus thrombosis, hypertension, and diabetes have been suggested as predisposing factors.[12,13] Trauma is less commonly associated with symptomatic indirect CCFs.[14] Congenital indirect CCFs have been reported in children, including infants as young as 5 weeks of age.[15]

The prevalence of types B, C, and D CCFs is uncertain: their frequency in a referral population is not representative of their occurrence in the general population.

CLINICAL PRESENTATION

The classic presentation for a direct, high-flow CCF is the sudden development of a clinical triad: exophthalmos, bruit, and conjunctival chemosis. Direct CCFs can develop following a traumatic tear of the cavernous segment of the ICA and/or rupture of a cavernous ICA aneurysm.[7,16,17] Complete disruption of the ICA wall allows highly pressurized arterial blood to be transmitted directly into the cavernous sinus and the ophthalmic veins, leading to venous hypertension. The manifestations of venous hypertension include ocular signs (**Fig. 1**) and symptoms (proptosis, chemosis, conjunctival injection, cranial nerve pareses, and visual deficits), bleeding (from mouth, nose, or ears), and cerebral complications (intracranial hemorrhage, increased intracranial pressure, and steal phenomena).[18,19] Five percent of patients develop intracranial hemorrhage, and 1% to 2% manifest life-threatening epistaxis. Epistaxis can be either acute or remote from the initial trauma caused by rupture of a pseudoaneurysmal cavernous sinus varix.

Compared with direct CCFs, indirect fistulas have a gradual onset, generally with a milder clinical presentation. Indirect fistulas usually are low-flow, acquired lesions that result from sinus thrombosis leading to venous congestion. Subsequently, abnormal arteriovenous shunting develops through the recanalized dural veins.[20] DAVFs of the cavernous sinus often do not demonstrate the classic triad of symptoms. Patients who have these fistulas have chronically red eyes because of tortuous arterialization of the conjunctival veins. An ocular bruit may or may not be present with these lesions.

Unlike direct high-flow fistulas, most spontaneous indirect DAVFs improve, and many heal with medical management.[21,22]

DIAGNOSTIC IMAGING

CT and MR imaging often are used in the initial work-up of a possible CCF. CT findings in CCFs include proptosis, enlargement of the extraocular muscles, enlargement and tortuosity of the superior ophthalmic vein, and enlargement of the ipsilateral cavernous sinus. MR imaging findings in CCFs are similar to those seen on CT with the addition of orbital edema and abnormal flow voids in the affected cavernous sinus.[23] In the setting of a high-flow fistula and retrograde cortical venous reflux, MR or CT studies may reveal dilatation of leptomeningeal and cortical veins. In patients who have cerebral venous congestion and elevated intracranial pressures, cerebral edema and/or hemorrhage may be encountered.

Digital subtraction angiography is essential in confirming the diagnosis, classifying the fistula, and delineating the venous drainage pathways. Specifically, conventional angiography best characterizes the flow rate of the fistula and clearly distinguishes between direct and indirect fistulas (exact anatomic location of ICA tear versus dural ICA/ECA feeders). Moreover, it helps to assess the draining venous pathways (anterior versus posterior), cortical venous reflux, venous stenosis, or occlusions that could limit transvenous access to the cavernous sinus.

A complete and detailed diagnostic angiogram is recommended for planning either endovascular or surgical treatment. Selective ICA and ECA

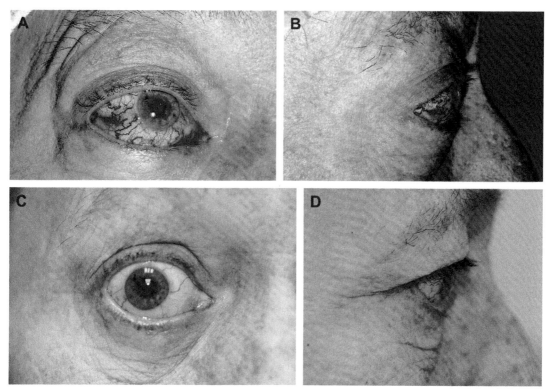

Fig. 1. (*A*, *B*) Photographs of a patient's eye before treatment of a traumatic, direct carotid cavernous fistula demonstrate proptosis, ptosis, chemosis, and arterialization of the conjunctival veins. (*C*, *D*) Same eye photographed after endovascular treatment demonstrates complete resolution of the clinical findings.

injections allow accurate classification of the fistula: direct fistula from the ICA or indirect dural fistula supplied by branches of the ICA/ECA. In addition, vertebral artery injections are helpful in fully appreciating the intracranial collateral circulation and circle of Willis in case ICA sacrifice must be considered as an option.

In evaluating direct CCFs, localizing the rent in the ICA can be challenging because of the high flow–related washout of intra-arterial contrast and instantaneous opacification of the cavernous sinus. Angiographic high-frame-rate imaging (> 5 frames/second) and rapid contrast injection rates (7 or 8 mL/second) may assist in evaluating the morphology of high-flow fistulas. If these techniques fail to identify the site of the fistulous communication accurately, specific maneuvers to decrease the flow rate across the fistula may be attempted. The Mehringer-Hieshima maneuver consists of injecting the ipsilateral ICA and manual compression of the ipsilateral common carotid artery while filming at a slower frame rate. Use of this maneuver slows the rate of opacification of the fistula and thereby allows better delineation of the fistula site. Another maneuver is the Huber maneuver, which involves injection of the

ipsilateral vertebral artery with manual compression of the affected carotid artery.[24] With this maneuver, the fistula is opacified through a posterior communicating artery if patent.

High-frame-rate imaging and magnified views of the head and neck allow detailed vascular mapping for anticipated transarterial and/or transvenous approaches. Delayed angiographic sequences incorporate the venous phase and help evaluate the patency of the major venous drainage pathways and the presence of cortical venous reflux and venous tortuosity and/or stenosis.

MEDICAL MANAGEMENT

Unlike high-flow direct CCFs, low-flow indirect or dural CCFs are not associated with increased mortality or significant risk for intracranial hemorrhage. Even in anterior draining fistulas that may lead to ocular manifestations, approximately 20% to 50% of dural CCFs heal spontaneously within days to months after symptomatic presentation. Therefore, an accepted practice is to treat the patient's ocular symptoms medically with prism therapy or patching for diplopia, topical agents for elevated intraocular pressure, lubrication for proptosis-related keratopathy, and/or systemic corticosteroids if needed.[25]

Furthermore, manual external carotid compression therapy may be initiated as a noninvasive treatment for indirect CCFs. This type of therapy is particularly effective in patients harboring fistulas in the anterior cavernous sinus and those who have relatively lower ocular pressures and a short interval between symptom onset and initiation of treatment.[26] The patient is instructed to sit in a chair or lie in bed, compressing the carotid artery and jugular vein with the contralateral hand for a period of 10 seconds, four to six times each hour. Intermittent self-administered manual carotid-jugular compression alone can result in a cure in 30% of patients.[21]

Contraindications to manual carotid compression include hypertensive carotid sinus syndrome, atherosclerotic stenosis, ulceration of the carotid artery, and a history of cerebral ischemia, because patients who have these anomalies cannot tolerate the transient occlusion of the ipsilateral ICA. The therapy must be discontinued if visual function shows progressive decline, the ocular pressure exceeds 25 mm Hg, or patients experience unbearable orbital pain.[26]

Signs of ocular morbidity alter a conservative medical approach toward surgical or endovascular intervention. Patients who have progressive visual decline, diplopia, optic disc edema refractory to medication, proliferative retinopathy, increasing intraocular pressures, headaches, intraparenchymal hemorrhage, angiographic evidence of retrograde (cortical) venous drainage, or significant cosmetic deformity resulting from the fistula are offered definitive endovascular treatment.[22]

SURGICAL TREATMENT

Early treatment for CCF consisted of various surgical approaches. Trapping of the fistula by ligation of the cervical and intracranial ICA was described in the 1930s. Alternatively, carotid sacrifice was performed via embolization using different materials delivered by direct carotid exposure.

Although surgical trapping with ligation of the ICA is still considered an effective treatment for direct CCFs, sacrifice of the ICA is performed sparingly because of a significant risk of cerebral infarction even after successful balloon test occlusion studies. Furthermore, endovascular treatment now can offer similar results with a less invasive approach, avoiding the difficult surgical drilling needed for exposure of the clinoidal segment of the ICA.

In 1974, Parkison[27] reported successful treatment of 9 of 11 patients by surgical exposure and packing of the cavernous sinus with preservation of the ICA. Although this surgical technique is useful for both direct and indirect CCFs, its role is limited if endovascular treatment can be performed because of its associated morbidity from cranial nerve deficits and residual fistulas.

Rarely, orbital surgery or decompression can be offered in cases that that do not respond to endovascular/surgical treatment or to those in which elevated intraocular pressures persist despite closure of the fistula.[25]

ENDOVASCULAR TREATMENT

Recent advances in endovascular technology have made a number of different treatment options for CCFs currently available. The exact method chosen in each case depends on the anatomy of the fistula and operator/institutional preferences (Fig. 2).

Direct fistulas occur from a tear in the cavernous segment of the ICA (Fig. 2A) or, less commonly, from the intracavernous rupture of an ICA aneurysm. The goal of treatment in direct CCFs is to occlude the site of communication between the ICA and the cavernous sinus while preserving the patency of the ICA. This goal can be accomplished with either transarterial obliteration of the fistula with a detachable balloon (Figs. 2B and 3), transarterial or transvenous obliteration of the ipsilateral cavernous sinus with coils or other embolic materials (Fig. 2C), or deployment of a covered stent across the fistula (Fig. 2D). Rarely, if the defect is large and cannot be repaired, the ICA may need to be sacrificed or trapped.

Indirect fistulas consist of small dural arteriovenous shunts between the meningeal branches of the ICA, the ECA, or both and the cavernous sinus. The goal of treatment in this condition is to interrupt the fistulous communications and decrease the pressure in the cavernous sinus. This goal can be accomplished by occluding the arterial branches supplying the fistula (transarterial embolization) or, more commonly, by occluding the cavernous sinus that harbors the fistulous communications (transvenous embolization).

The following sections provide a brief overview of the various endovascular options for the treatment of CCFs.

Transarterial Methods

In 1974, Serbinenko[28] reported the first case of successful embolization of a CCF from an endovascular approach using a detachable balloon. Subsequently, Debrun and colleagues[29] reported

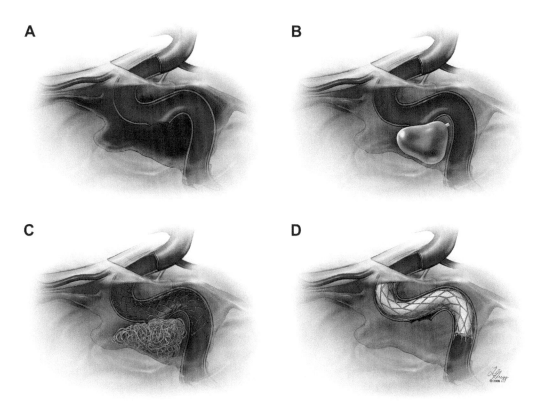

Fig. 2. Artist's rendition of a direct CCF. (*A*) The tear in the proximal horizontal cavernous segment of the internal carotid artery is shown with direct communication to a distended cavernous sinus. (*B*) Detachable balloon embolization is an elegant and effective option for the treatment. The balloon (shown in blue) is floated across the fistula and is inflated against the defect in the artery. (*C*) Stent-assisted coil embolization of direct CCF: schematic diagram of placement of an intracranial porous stent across the arterial defect and closure of the fistula with detachable coils. (*D*) An alternative option for endovascular management is to cover the arterial defect with a covered stent graft. These stents are relatively stiff and therefore are difficult to use when proximal arterial tortuosity is present. (*Courtesy of* L. Gregg, Baltimore, MD; with permission. Copyright © Lydia Gregg 2009.)

their successful treatment in 12 of 17 patients using detachable balloons. By the 1980s, detachable balloons were widely accepted as the treatment of choice for direct CCFs, although most balloons used in the United States were imported from abroad. The Food and Drug Administration (FDA) approved a detachable balloon system for peripheral vessel occlusion in 1981, but problems with the detachment system led to its withdrawal from the market in 1991. The first FDA-approved detachable balloon for intracranial use was not approved until 1998. Unfortunately, the balloon was removed from the United States market in 2003 because of problems with the valve mechanism, however, it continues to be available in many other parts of the world, however.

If available, the ideal treatment for a high-flow, direct CCF remains transarterial obliteration of the fistula with a detachable balloon.[30,31] The balloon offers the advantage of being able to be flow-directed through the fistula and into the

cavernous sinus. The balloon is inflated to a volume larger than the orifice of the fistula to prevent its retrograde prolapse into the ICA and then is detached. This approach constitutes an inexpensive, simple, but elegant endovascular treatment for direct CCFs (see **Figs. 2**B and **3**).

Occasionally, technical problems have been encountered with detachable balloon embolization, such as failure of flow-directed advancement from the ICA into the cavernous sinus or difficulty passing the balloon through the rent in the ICA. Additionally, early detachment/deflation of the balloon and occasional rupture of the balloon caused by contact with bone fragments have occurred.[7,32]

Transarterial embolization with coils or other embolic material now is the mainstay of endovascular treatment for high-flow direct CCFs, given the unavailability of detachable balloons. Commonly used embolic agents include detachable platinum coils, n-butyl cyanoacrylate

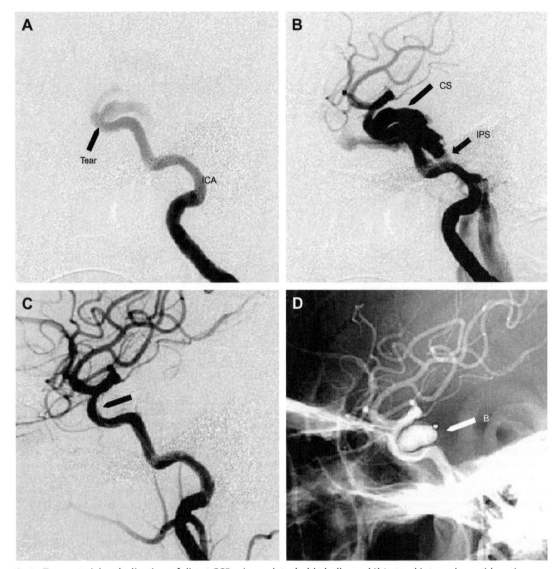

Fig. 3. Transarterial embolization of direct CCF using a detachable balloon. (*A*) Lateral internal carotid angiogram, early arterial phase, demonstrates a tear (*arrow*) within the cavernous segment of the internal carotid artery (ICA) resulting in a high-flow direct CCF. (*B*) Later arterial phase of this angiogram shows rapid shunting of contrast into the cavernous sinus (CS) and inferior petrosal sinus (IPS). (*C*) Lateral internal carotid angiogram after detachable balloon placement in the cavernous sinus. Arrow demonstrates occlusion of the arterial tear and the CC. (*D*) Nonsubtracted image of lateral internal carotid angiogram shown in panel C shows the detachable balloon (B) in the cavernous sinus. (*Courtesy of* N.K. Mishra, MD, Lausanne, Switzerland. *From* Gemmete J, Ansari SA, Gandhi D. Endovascular techniques for treatment of carotid-cavernous fistula. J Neuro Opthalmol 2009;29(1):62–71; with permission.)

(n-BCA), and ethylene-vinyl alcohol copolymer (EVOH).

The standard transarterial approach consists of placing a guiding catheter in the cervical ICA. Next, a microcatheter is superselectively advanced into the cavernous segment of the ICA and across the tear into the cavernous sinus. Through this microcatheter, embolic material is placed into the cavernous sinus.

The authors prefer to use detachable platinum coils because of their reliable and controlled deployment. The coils can be adjusted easily or even removed if the placement is not optimal.[33] The use of transarterial liquid embolic agents such as n-BCA or EVOH to occlude direct CCFs also have been described.[34,35] During transarterial embolization, a temporary balloon may be placed in the cavernous segment of the ICA (across the site of the tear) to protect the parent vessel and to prevent migration of the embolic material into the distal intracranial circulation.

CCFs caused by a small tear in the ICA can be treated with detachable balloons or coils as described. If there is a fairly large rent in the artery, however, the coils or balloon may herniate (or migrate) through the defect into the parent vessel. This retrograde herniation of embolic material can cause vessel occlusion and thromboembolic complications.

Recently, dedicated, intracranial, self-expanding stents have become available. These stents are approved by the FDA for coil embolization of wide-necked intracranial aneurysms. In the setting of direct CCFs, however, they can provide valuable scaffolding to reconstruct a severely injured intracranial ICA (see Fig. 2C).

When deployed across a traumatic tear, stents create a barrier between the ICA and the cavernous sinus, preventing retrograde herniation of coils into the parent artery.[36] These devices allow initial reconstruction of the damaged segment of the ICA and then controlled deposition of coils into the cavernous sinus through either a transarterial or transvenous approach. Using this technique, a direct CCF with severe injury to the ICA now can be occluded while preserving the ICA.

Direct CCFs caused by extensive injury to the ICA may not be amenable to endovascular occlusion with preservation of the parent artery. In these cases, occlusion of the arterial segment bearing the fistula may be the only viable option for treatment. If time permits, and the patient is cooperative, a temporary balloon test occlusion study of the involved ICA is recommended before permanent occlusion. Some risk of ischemic complications remain after ICA sacrifice despite a successful balloon test occlusion study.

To prevent retrograde flow from the supraclinoid ICA into the fistula, vessel occlusion is initiated cranial to the site of the suspected tear. Using multiple coils, the cavernous ICA then is occluded at the level of and caudal to the site of the fistula. This technique may be life saving in a patient who has extensive and unstable injuries. Recently, hydrogel-coated detachable coils have been introduced that expand on contact with blood, a favorable property especially in resilient high-flow fistulas that require high volumetric packing of the cavernous sinus. Furthermore, these coils may facilitate vessel sacrifice, decreasing the procedure and fluoroscopy times.[37] Use of a vascular plug for arterial sacrifice also has been reported.[38] Although the plug is easy to deploy and is effective,

the navigation of the vascular plug into the distal ICA is currently difficult.

Placement of a stent or graft covered with polyfluorotetraethylene is an alternative treatment option if ICA sacrifice is not desired or is unacceptable because of an unsuccessful balloon test occlusion study (Figs. 2D and 4). Covered stent grafts can be extremely useful for the immediate obliteration of a direct CCF and other fistulas. Additionally, they may decrease the risk of ischemic stroke by preserving the involved artery while simultaneously sealing the site of the fistula. A few reports have described the successful use of a covered stent graft for the treatment of CCFs.[39–41] Currently, the FDA has not approved any covered stent for intracranial use in the United States. The disadvantages of the stents include stiff and high-profile construction that make it difficult to navigate them into the distal ICA, risk of endoleaks, possibility of coverage of vital perforators, and lack of long-term safety data.

Transarterial embolization of indirect low-flow CCFs generally is cumbersome because of the small size, tortuous anatomy, and multiplicity of arterial feeders. The transvenous approach often is simpler and carries a high rate of success. The venous approach may fail in a small percentage of patients, however; in these cases, transarterial embolization still can be a viable alternative.

Transarterial techniques involve distal catheterization of the small meningeal branches supplying the fistula. Ideally, superselective microcatheter placement is performed with microcatheter tip as close as possible to the point of fistulous communication. Once a satisfactory microcatheter position is achieved, liquid embolic agents are injected under fluoroscopic control with the goal of occluding the fistulous connections and penetrating the cavernous sinus. Although coils and particulate agents have been used, these agents used alone cannot cause permanent occlusion of the fistula.

The most commonly used agent for transarterial embolization is n-BCA glue, a monomeric liquid adhesive approved in the United States for use in presurgical embolization of cerebral arteriovenous malformations.[42] The viscosity and polymerization time of n-BCA is controlled by the addition of Lipiodol. The advantages of n-BCA include its thrombogenic nature and permanent occlusion of the injected feeders. Drawbacks of this agent include its rapid polymerization time (a few seconds), adhesive nature (risk of catheter retention), and a relatively long learning curve for its optimal use.

EVOH is another useful liquid embolic agent, recently approved by the FDA for the preoperative embolization of brain arteriovenous

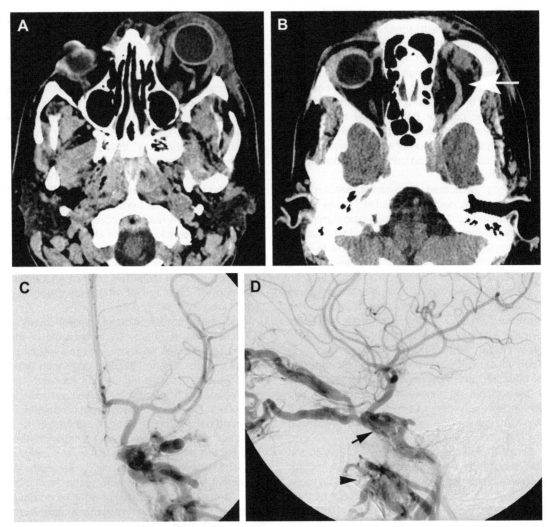

Fig. 4. High-flow, posttraumatic CCF treated by a combination of transarterial and transvenous approaches. (*A, B*) Axial CT scan demonstrates proptosis, preseptal edema, and a dilated SOV (*arrow*). (*C*) Anteroposterior and (*D*) lateral left internal carotid angiograms from the same patient. Note the high-flow direct CCF from a tear within the cavernous segment of the ICA filling the cavernous sinus (*arrow*), SOV, and pterygoid venous plexus (*arrowhead*). (*E*) Spot fluoroscopic image during the placement of a covered stent within the cavernous segment of the ICA (*arrows*). (*F*) Control angiogram from the same patient after placement of a covered stent in the cavernous segment reveals significantly reduced opacification of the fistula. Slight residual shunting remained even after the placement of this stent, however. (*G*) The residual fistula was obliterated via coil embolization (arrows identify the subtraction artifact caused by the coils) of the cavernous sinus using a transvenous IPS approach. This final control angiogram shows complete closure of the fistula.

malformations, that also may be used for transarterial embolization of indirect CCFs. EVOH is a nonadhesive liquid embolic agent with a lavalike flow pattern. It is supplied in ready-to-use vials with mixture of EVOH, dimethyl sulfoxide solvent (DMSO), and tantalum. Currently 6% and 8% EVOH concentrations (dissolved in DMSO) are available in the United States. When the mixture contacts aqueous media, such as blood, DMSO rapidly diffuses away from the mixture causing in-situ precipitation, solidification of the polymer,

and the formation of a spongy embolus. Polymerization occurs more slowly than with n-BCA, and because EVOH is nonadherent to the walls of the vessel or microcatheter, it allows prolonged injection times while decreasing the chances of permanent microcatheter retention. Because of the slower polymerization times, the ability to make controlled injections over minutes, and the ability to direct and push the embolic agent into the desired location, the use of EVOH may allow better and more distal penetration of the nidus or fistula

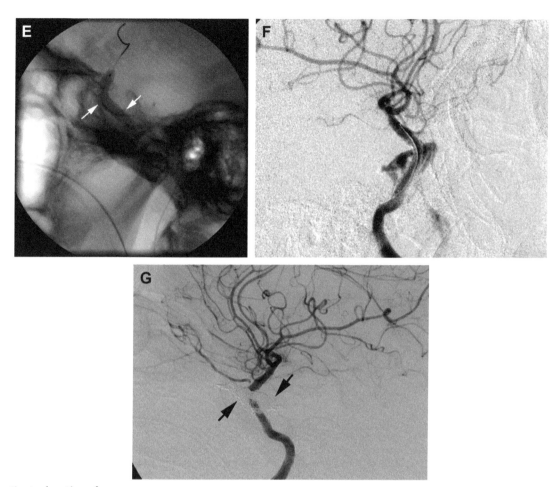

Fig. 4. (continued)

than possible with n-BCA. EVOH offers the possibility of venous sinus packing/occlusion using a transarterial approach, an advantage that may be quite helpful in cases in which venous access to the cavernous sinus is limited because of stenosis or occlusion of the major draining venous pathways (Fig. 5). The authors recently have reported the successful use of transarterial embolization of an indirect CCF using EVOH to occlude the cavernous sinus.[43]

Conversely, some concern for residual intraluminal flow following EVOH embolization remains because of the cohesive, nonadherent, and laminar properties of the agent. Additionally, the risk of penetration into ECA supply to the cranial nerves or retrograde reflux into ECA-ICA collaterals may be greater with prolonged EVOH injections. Further difficulties in the transarterial treatment of indirect CCFs are related to the small size and tortuousity of vessels supplying the fistula. Superselective distal access into these tiny feeders often is difficult or impossible, and multiple staged sessions may be necessary.

Transvenous Methods

Transvenous embolization has become the preferred method of treatment for indirect CCFs. Moreover, it may be an option in direct CCFs that cannot be treated by a transarterial route because of inaccessibility of the proximal ICA secondary to traumatic injury, severe tortuosity, and/or inability to catheterize the ICA tear.

For indirect CCFs the authors first attempt transvenous techniques because of their simplicity in comparison to transarterial methods, the frequent ability to cure the fistula in a single session, and the high rate of success. The aim of treatment is to catheterize the abnormal cavernous sinus superselectively and to occlude this sinus using embolic agents.

The most commonly used venous pathway for cannulation of the cavernous sinuses is via the inferior petrosal sinus (IPS) (Fig. 6). This transvenous route usually is from a posterior approach through the internal jugular vein and the IPS up to the pathologic shunts of the cavernous sinus.[44]

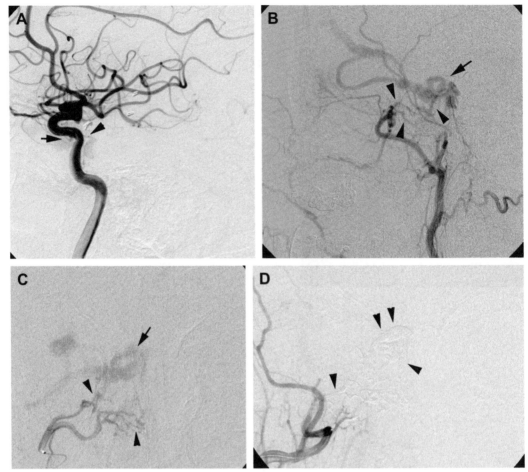

Fig. 5. Indirect type D CCF presenting with right-sided proptosis, chemosis, and periorbital edema. (*A*) Right ICA angiogram, lateral view, reveals inferolateral trunk (*arrow*) and meningohypophyseal trunk (*arrowhead*) minimally opacifying the cavernous sinus. (*B*) Lateral view of right external carotid angiogram demonstrating multiple small arterial feeders (*arrowheads*) from the right internal maxillary artery filling a septated, irregular cavernous sinus. The inferior petrosal, superior petrosal, and the circular sinus were occluded. Although the SOV was patent, a severe stenosis at the junction of the SOV with the angular vein prevented its catheterization. (*C*) Multiple attempts were made to catheterize the cavernous sinus without any success. Subsequently, a microcatheter was placed in the right internal maxillary artery, and an angiogram was performed via the microcatheter (anteroposterior view shown here). The CCF feeders are indicated by arrowheads and the cavernous sinus by an arrow. (*D*) The CCF was embolized with EVOH via a transarterial approach. The EVOH penetrated from the distal internal maxillary artery into the arterial branches feeding the fistula and subsequently into the cavernous sinus. This postembolization control angiogram of the right ECA demonstrates complete occlusion of the fistula. The EVOH cast is seen here as a subtraction artifact (*arrowheads*).

If the IPS is occluded or absent, access into the cavernous sinus can be obtained from an anterior approach through the superior ophthalmic vein (SOV) via the facial vein.[45] Other percutaneous transvenous approaches include the pterygoid venous plexus, superior petrosal sinus, cortical veins, or the contralateral IPS or SOV with access into the ipsilateral cavernous sinus through the circular sinus.[46,47]

Alternatively, in extremely difficult cases of venous occlusion, stenosis, or marked tortuosity, combined surgical and endovascular approaches may be needed to access the cavernous sinus. Direct transorbital puncture or indirect puncture through the superior or inferior ophthalmic vein

(SOV/IOV) allows straightforward access to the cavernous sinus.[48] Surgical access also may be obtained into the SOV, superficial middle cerebral vein, or sphenoparietal sinus leading to the cavernous sinus. Following catheterization of the cavernous sinus, disconnection of the venous outflow from the feeding arteries at the level of the fistula can be initiated with detachable coils (**Fig. 7**) or liquid embolic agents.

Embolic materials include coils, n-BCA, and EVOH, can be used either alone or in combination. Again, the advantages of coils include their radiopacity, ease of use, and the ability to redeploy or remove the devices if the initial placement is not optimal. However, there may be difficulty in

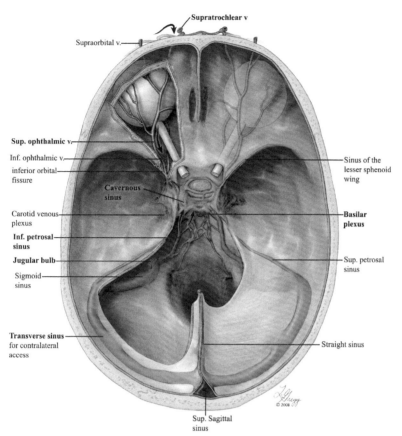

Fig. 6. An artist's rendition of the skull base dural sinuses looking from above demonstrates multiple possible pathways to again access into the cavernous sinus for transvenous occlusion of a CCF. If the inferior petrosal sinus is patent, it provides a relatively straightforward access to the cavernous sinus. Other access routes include the SOV, IOV, superior petrosal sinus, and the basilar venous plexus. (*Courtesy of* L. Gregg, Baltimore, MD; with permission. Copyright © Lydia Gregg 2009.)

achieving adequate volumetric packing or complete occlusion, especially in septated cavernous sinuses. Moreover, the reported rates of cranial nerve paresis are higher with coil embolization, probably because of their mass effect.

Consequently, transvenous liquid embolic agents are being used increasingly, either alone or in combination with platinum coils.[49,50] Liquid embolic agents can readily permeate different sinus compartments, allowing complete occlusion of the fistula. In a series of 14 patients in which n-BCA was used either alone or in conjunction with coils, Wakhloo and colleagues[49] reported the technique to be safe and effective for the treatment of complex indirect CCFs in symptomatic patients.

As described earlier, EVOH is a new liquid embolic agent that may be used in the transvenous embolization of direct or indirect CCFs. At this time, only a few case reports describe the successful transvenous treatment of indirect CCFs with EVOH.[50] It must be remembered that EVOH has a propensity for retrograde filling of arterial feeders and must be used cautiously. The inadvertent penetration of EVOH into ECA branches supplying the cranial nerves can potentially result in cranial nerve paralysis. Similarly, there is the potential for EVOH to migrate into the meningeal branches of the ICA and thereby reflux retrogradely into the ICA. Therefore, careful attention should be paid to the EVOH cast as the embolization progresses. Control angiograms should be performed if there is any doubt regarding reflux of this agent into the arterial feeders supplying the fistula. Given its favorable properties, EVOH probably will be used more widely in the future for the transvenous treatment of CCFs.

Endovascular Outcomes

The reported success rate of detachable balloon embolizations for direct CCFs is 88% to

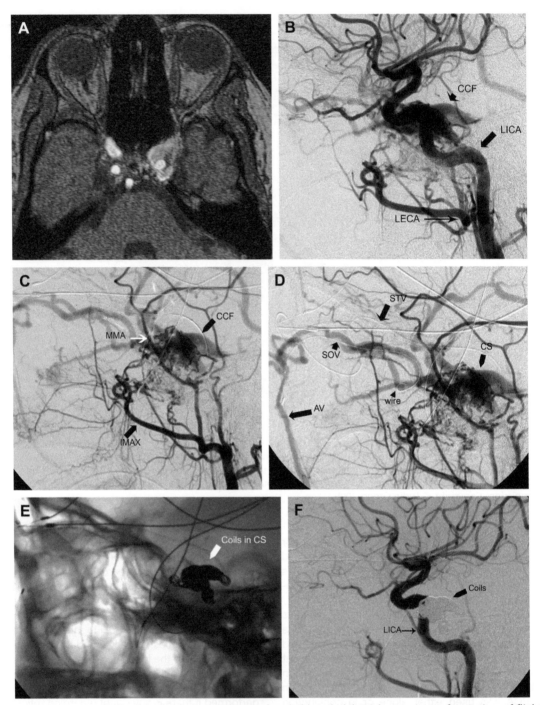

Fig. 7. Transvenous embolization of an indirect CCF using detachable coils. (*A*) Axial source image from a time-of-flight MR angiographic image reveals an enlarged left cavernous sinus, a finding consistent with a clinically known CCF. (*B*) Lateral view of the left common carotid angiogram confirms a type D CCF, filling from the meningeal branches of the left ICA (LICA) and left ECA (LECA). (*C*) Lateral view of the selective left external carotid angiogram demonstrates the branches of the internal maxillary artery (IMAX) and the middle meningeal artery (MMA) contributing to the CCF. (*D*) The inferior and superior petrosal sinuses as well the circular sinus were occluded in this patient. The SOV was catheterized via superficial temporal vein (STV), and access to the cavernous sinus was obtained. This lateral view of the left external carotid angiogram demonstrates the microwire at the confluence of the left SOV and the cavernous sinus (CS). The microwire courses through the STV and the SOV. AV denotes the angular vein. (*E*) Lateral projection shows detachable coils within the left cavernous sinus (CS). (*F*) Lateral view of a left common carotid angiogram (LCCA) after coil embolization of the cavernous sinus demonstrates complete occlusion of the CCF.

99%.[6,7,51] Kobayashi and colleagues[52] achieved 80% aneurysmal and 55% posttraumatic CCF closure with a detachable balloon. Higashida and colleagues[6] treated more than 200 traumatic CCFs, achieving complete occlusion of the fistula in 99% of patients and preserving the parent artery in 88% of patients. Gupta and colleagues[53] achieved complete occlusion in 86.3% of fistulas, nearly total occlusion in 11.0%, and ICA preservation in 98%. The percentage of patients experiencing morbidity associated with embolizations of direct CCFs, such as ICA occlusion or worsening of ocular palsy, has ranged from 10% to 40%.[7,50,54,55]

The reported complete cure rate for indirect CCFs is 70% to 90% with a complication rate of 2.3% to 5%.[22,56-58] Meyers and colleagues[58] reported on endovascular treatment and clinical outcome in 135 patients who had indirect CCFs over a 15-year period. Endovascular treatment was performed in 133 patients (98%), and clinical follow-up was available in all 135 patients (mean duration of follow-up 56 ± 4.3 months). Angiographic follow-up was performed in 72 patients (54%) who had ongoing symptoms or a history of fistula with high-risk angiographic features. At a mean follow-up of 56 months, 121 patients (90%) were clinically cured. The rate of procedure-related permanent morbidity was 2.3%. There was no operative mortality.

ACKNOWLEDGMENTS

The authors thank Lydia Gregg, BFA, MA, medical illustrator and research associate, Division of Interventional Neuroradiology, Johns Hopkins University, for the anatomic illustrations presented in this article.

REFERENCES

1. Barrow DL, Spector RH, Braun IF, et al. Classification and treatment of spontaneous carotid-cavernous sinus fistulas. J Neurosurg 1985;62(2):248–56.
2. Locke CE. Intracranial arteriovenous aneurism or pulsating exophthalmos. Ann Surg 1924;80(1):1–24.
3. Tomsick TA. Type A (direct) CCF: etiology, prevalence, and natural history. In: Tomsick T, editor. Carotid cavernous fistula. Cincinnati (OH): Digital Educational Publishing; 1997. p. 35–8.
4. Debrun G, Lacour P, Vinuela F, et al. Treatment of 54 carotid-cavernous fistulas. J Neurosurg 1981;55(5):678–92.
5. Van Dellen JR. Intracavernous traumatic aneurysms. Surg Neurol 1980;13(3):203–7.
6. Higashida RT, Halbach VV, Tsai FY, et al. Interventional neurovascular treatment of traumatic carotid and vertebral lesions: results in 234 cases. AJR Am J Roentgenol 1989;153(3):577–82.
7. Lewis AI, Tomsick TA, Tew JM. Management of 100 consecutive direct carotid-cavernous fistulas: results of treatment with detachable balloons. Neurosurgery 1995;36(2):239–44.
8. Gossman MD, Berlin AJ, Weinstein MA, et al. Spontaneous direct carotid-cavernous fistula in childhood. Ophthal Plast Reconstr Surg 1993;9(1):62–5.
9. Debrun G, Vinuela F, Fox AJ, et al. Indications for treatment and classification of 132 carotid-cavernous fistulas. Neurosurgery 1988;22(2):285–9.
10. Hieshima GB, Cahan LD, Mehringer CM, et al. Spontaneous arteriovenous fistulas of cerebral vessels in association with fibromuscular dysplasia. Neurosurgery 1986;18(4):454–8.
11. Kashiwaga S, Tsuchida E, Goto K, et al. Balloon occlusion of spontaneous carotid-cavernous fistula in Ehlers-Danlos syndrome type IV. Surg Neurol 1993;39(3):187–90.
12. Houser OW, Campbell JK, Campbell RJ, et al. Arteriovenous malformation affecting the transverse dural venous sinus—an acquired lesion. Mayo Clin Proc 1979;54(10):651–61.
13. Graeb DA, Dolman CL. Radiological and pathological aspects of dural arteriovenous fistulas: case report. J Neurosurg 1986;64(6):962–7.
14. Komiyama M, Nakajima H, Nishikawa M, et al. Traumatic carotid cavernous sinus fistula: serial angiography studies from the day of trauma. AJNR Am J Neuroradiol 1998;19(9):1641–4.
15. Pang D, Kerber C, Biglan AW, et al. External carotid-cavernous fistula in infancy: case report and review of the literature. Neurosurgery 1981;8(2):212–8.
16. Halbach VV, Higashida RT, Hieshima GB, et al. Transvenous embolization of direct carotid cavernous fistulas. AJNR Am J Neuroradiol 1988;9(4):741–7.
17. D'Angelo VA, Monte V, Scialfa G, et al. Intracerebral venous hemorrhage in "high risk" carotid-cavernous fistula. Surg Neurol 1988;30(5):387–90.
18. Vinuela F, Fox AJ, Debrun GM, et al. Spontaneous carotid-cavernous fistulas: clinical, radiological, and therapeutic considerations: experience with 20 cases. J Neurosurg 1984;60(5):976–84.
19. Halbach VV, Hieshima GB, Higashida RT, et al. Carotid cavernous fistulae: indications for urgent treatment. AJR Am J Roentgenol 1987;149(3):587–93.
20. Kwan E, Hieshima GB, Higashida RT, et al. Interventional neuroradiology in neuro-ophthalmology. J Clin Neuroophthalmol 1989;9(2):83–97.
21. Higashida RT, Hieshima GB, Halbach VV, et al. Closure of carotid cavernous sinus fistulae by external compression of the carotid artery and jugular vein. Acta Radiol Suppl 1986;369:580–3.

22. Halbach VV, Higashida RT, Hieshima GB, et al. Dural fistulas involving the cavernous sinus: Results of treatment in 30 patients. Radiology 1987;163(2): 437–42.

23. Elster AD, Chen MY, Richardson DN, et al. Dilated intercavernous sinuses: an MR sign of carotid-cavernous and carotid-dural fistulas. AJNR Am J Neuroradiol 1991;12(4):641–5.

24. Huber P. A technical contribution to the exact angiographic localization of carotid cavernous fistulas. Neuroradiology 1976;10(5):239–41.

25. Miller NR. Diagnosis and management of dural carotid-cavernous sinus fistulas. Neurosurg Focus 2007;23(5):E13.

26. Kai Y, Hamada J, Morioka M, et al. Treatment of cavernous sinus dural arteriovenous fistulae by external manual carotid compression. Neurosurgery 2007;60(2):253–7 [discussion: 257–8].

27. Parkison D, Downs AR, Whytehead LL, et al. Carotid cavernous fistula: direct repair with preservation of carotid. Surgery 1975;76(6):882–9.

28. Serbinenko FA. Balloon catheterization and occlusion of major cerebral vessels. J Neurosurg 1974; 41(2):125–45.

29. Debrun G, Lacour P, Caron JP, et al. Detachable balloon and calibrated-leak balloon techniques in the treatment of cerebral vascular lesions. J Neurosurg 1978;49(5):635–49.

30. Goto K, Hieshima GB, Higashida RT, et al. Treatment of direct carotid cavernous sinus fistulae. Various therapeutic approaches and results in 148 cases. Acta Radiol Suppl 1986;369:576–9.

31. Teng MM, Chang CY, Chiang JH, et al. Double-balloon technique for embolization of carotid cavernous fistulas. AJNR Am J Neuroradiol 2000; 21(9):1753–6.

32. Norman D, Newton TH, Edwards MSB. Carotid cavernous fistula: closure with detachable silicone balloon. Radiology 1983;149(1):149–59.

33. Halbach VV, Higashida RT, Barnwell SL, et al. Transarterial platinum coil embolization of carotid-cavernous fistulas. AJNR Am J Neuroradiol 1991; 12(3):429–33.

34. Lv XL, Li YX, Liu AH, et al. A complex cavernous sinus dural arteriovenous fistula secondary to covered stent placement for a traumatic carotid artery-cavernous sinus fistula: case report. J Neurosurg 2008;108(3):588–90.

35. Luo CB, Teng MM, Chang FC, et al. Transarterial balloon-assisted n-butyl-2-cyanoacrylate embolization of direct carotid cavernous fistulas. AJNR Am J Neuroradiol 2006;27(7):1535–40.

36. Moron FE, Klucznik RP, Mawad ME, et al. Endovascular treatment of high flow carotid cavernous fistula by stent-assisted coil placement. AJNR Am J Neuroradiol 2005;26(6):1399–404.

37. Kallmes DF, Cloft HJ. The use of hydrocoil for parent vessel occlusion. AJNR Am J Neuroradiol 2004; 25(8):1409–10.

38. Ross IB, Buciuc R. The vascular plug: a new device for parent artery occlusion. AJNR Am J Neuroradiol 2007;28(2):385–6.

39. Madan A, Mujic A, Daniels K, et al. Traumatic carotid-cavernous sinus fistula treated with a covered stent. Report of two cases. J Neurosurg 2006;104(6):969–73.

40. Felber S, Henkes H, Weber W, et al. Treatment of extracranial and intracranial aneurysms and arteriovenous fistulae using stent grafts. Neurosurgery 2004;55(3):631–8 [discussion: 638–9].

41. Gomez F, Escobar W, Gomez AM, et al. Treatment of carotid cavernous fistulas using covered stents: midterm results in seven patients. AJNR Am J Neuroradiol 2007;28(9):1762–8.

42. Nelson PK, Russell SM, Woo HH, et al. Use of a wedged microcatheter for curative transarterial embolization of complex intracranial dural arteriovenous fistulas: indications, endovascular technique, and outcome in 21 patients. J Neurosurg 2003; 98(3):498–506.

43. Gandhi D, Ansari SA, Cornblath WT. Successful transarterial embolization of a Barrow type D dural carotid-cavernous fistula with ethylene vinyl alcohol copolymer (Onyx). J Neuro Opthalmol 2009;29(1): 9–12.

44. Klisch J, Huppertz HJ, Spetzger U, et al. Transvenous treatment of carotid cavernous and dural arteriovenous fistulae: results for 31 patients and review of the literature. Neurosurgery 2003;53(4): 836–56.

45. Biondi A, Milea D, Cognard C, et al. Cavernous sinus dural fistulae treated by transvenous approach through the facial vein: report of seven cases and review of the literature. AJNR Am J Neuroradiol 2003;24(6):1240–6.

46. Mounayer C, Piotin M, Spelle L, et al. Superior petrosal sinus catheterization for transvenous embolization of a dural carotid cavernous sinus fistula. AJNR Am J Neuroradiol 2002;23(7):1153–5.

47. Jahan R, Gobin YP, Glenn B, et al. Transvenous embolization of a dural arteriovenous fistula of the cavernous sinus through the contralateral pterygoid plexus. Neuroradiology 1998;40(3):189–93.

48. White JB, Layton KF, Evans AJ, et al. Transorbital puncture for the treatment of cavernous sinus dural arteriovenous fistulas. AJNR Am J Neuroradiol 2007;28(7):1415–7.

49. Wakhloo AK, Perlow A, Linfante I, et al. Transvenous n-butyl-cyanoacrylate infusion for complex dural carotid cavernous fistulas: technical considerations and clinical outcome. AJNR Am J Neuroradiol 2005;26(8):1888–97.

50. Suzuki S, Lee DW, Jahan R, et al. Transvenous treatment of spontaneous dural carotid-cavernous fistulas using a combination of detachable coils and Onyx. AJNR Am J Neuroradiol 2006;27(6):1346–9.

51. Debrun G, Lacour P, Vinuela F, et al. Treatment of 54 traumatic carotid-cavernous fistulas. J Neurosurg 1981;55(5):678–92.

52. Kobayashi N, Miyachi S, Negoro M, et al. Endovascular treatment strategy for direct carotid-cavernous fistulas resulting from rupture of intracavernous carotid aneurysms. AJNR Am J Neuroradiol 2003; 24(9):1789–96.

53. Gupta AK, Purkayasta S, Krishnamoorthy T, et al. Endovascular treatment of direct carotid cavernous fistulae: a pictorial review. Neuroradiology 2006; 48(11):831–9.

54. Klisch K, Schipper J, Husstedt H, et al. Transsphenoidal computer-navigation-assisted deflation of a balloon after endovascular occlusion of a direct carotid cavernous sinus fistula. AJNR Am J Neuroradiol 2001;22(3):537–40.

55. Halbach VV, Higashida RT, Dowd CF, et al. Treatment of carotid cavernous fistulas associated with Ehlers-Danlos syndrome. Neurosurgery 1990;26(6): 1021–7.

56. Picard L, Bracard S, Mallet J, et al. Spontaneous dural arteriovenous fistulas. Seminars in Interventional Radiology 1987;4:219–40.

57. Turjman F, Bascoulergue Y, Rosenberg M, et al. Dural fistulae of the cavernous sinus treated with embolization. Ten cases. J Neuroradiol 1992;19(4): 256–70.

58. Meyers PM, Halbach VV, Dowd CF, et al. Dural carotid cavernous fistula: definitive endovascular management and long-term follow-up. Am J Ophthalmol 2002;134(1):85–92.

Cervical Dissections: Diagnosis, Management, and Endovascular Treatment

Sameer A. Ansari, MD, PhD[a],*, Hemant Parmar, MD[b],
Mohannad Ibrahim, MD[b], Joseph J. Gemmete, MD[b],
Dheeraj Gandhi, MD[c]

KEYWORDS

- Cervical dissection • Dissecting aneurysm • Diagnosis
- Imaging • Management • Endovascular treatment
- Stent reconstruction

PATHOGENESIS AND EPIDEMIOLOGY

Cervical dissections result from intimal injury, laceration of the arterial wall or spontaneous hemorrhage of the vasa vasorum causing a subintimal or intramural hematoma. Although dissections may remain asymptomatic, mass effect from the subintimal false vascular channel or intramural hematoma can narrow the true vessel lumen ranging from minimal compromise to turbulent and impaired flow across the stenotic segment. Severe dissections may ultimately progress to complete vessel occlusion. If antegrade flow persists in the false lumen, it is termed a "double-barrel" dissection with parallel patent lumens converging distally into the true lumen. If an intramural hematoma expands peripherally into the tunica media and subadventitial space, dissecting aneurysms or pseudoaneurysms may develop with inflow/outflow zones communicating by way of the true lumen.

The incidence of spontaneous cervical (carotid/vertebral) dissections is low with approximately three to five cases per 100,000, but they contribute to as many as 10% to 20% of thromboembolic strokes in young and middle-age patients. Although there is a peak incidence in the fifth decade of life with comparatively younger female presentations, there is no definite sex predilection.[1]

Spontaneous etiologies are thought to be related to an inherent arteriopathy caused by genetic factors and connective tissue disorders such as Ehlers-Danlos syndrome type IV, Marfan syndrome, autosomal dominant polycystic kidney disease, osteogenesis imperfecta type I, and fibromuscular dysplasia (responsible for approximately 15% of spontaneous dissections). In addition, spontaneous dissections are associated with intracranial aneurysms, coarctation of the aorta, bicuspid aortic valve, a widened aortic root, arterial redundancy and distensibility. Using skin biopsy samples, Brandt and colleagues[2] demonstrated structural abnormalities in the extracellular matrix of subjects with spontaneous dissections, analogous to the collagen and elastic fiber abnormalities in patients with Ehlers-Danlos and Marfan syndromes respectively, suggesting underlying collagen vascular disease.[1–3]

[a] Departments of Radiology, Neurology, and Surgery, University of Chicago Medical Center, 5841 S. Maryland Avenue, MC-2026, Chicago, IL 60637, USA
[b] Department of Radiology, University of Michigan Health System, 1500 East Medical Center Drive, B1D330A, Ann Arbor, MI 48109, USA
[c] Johns Hopkins University and Hospitals, Departments of Radiology, Neurology, and Neurosurgery, Division of Interventional Neuroradiology, 600 N Wolfe St/Radiology B-100, Baltimore, MD 21287, USA
* Corresponding author. Departments of Radiology, Neurology, and Surgery, University of Chicago Medical Center, 5841 S. Maryland Avenue, MC-2026, Chicago, IL 60637.
E-mail address: sansari1@uchicago.edu (S.A. Ansari).

Neuroimag Clin N Am 19 (2009) 257–270
doi:10.1016/j.nic.2009.01.007
1052-5149/09/$ – see front matter © 2009 Elsevier Inc. All rights reserved.

Traumatic and iatrogenic dissections are predominantly due to blunt or penetrating injuries, chiropractic manipulation, or catheter angiography. The extracranial cervical arteries may be more susceptible to traumatic injury due to their mobility within the neck soft tissues along the cervical spine and tethering at the skull base; hence, the potential for direct injury from the adjacent bony structures.[1]

CLINICAL PRESENTATION

Patients with cervical dissections present after minor or major inciting events resulting in neck hyperextension or rotation, often with sudden transitional or decelerating movements. Although dissections can occur following major head and neck trauma associated with motor vehicle accidents, many patients have a history of more subtle trauma such as practicing yoga, painting a ceiling, coughing, vomiting, sneezing, recent catheter angiography, anesthesia or resuscitation. In particular, chiropractic manipulation is notorious for causing carotid, and more frequently, vertebral artery dissections with 1 in 20,000 manipulations resulting in stroke.[1,4]

Internal carotid artery dissections may present with the classic triad of ipsilateral headache or neck pain, partial Horner's syndrome, and ischemic symptoms. However, lower cranial nerve palsies (particularly the hypoglossal nerve), impairment of taste (facial and glossopharyngeal nerve palsies), pulsatile tinnitus (or auscultation of a bruit), and cerebral and retinal transient ischemic attacks or infarcts can also be present at the time of initial presentation.[1]

Nearly two thirds of patients with carotid dissections present with neck pain or headache usually described as a gradual onset of constant dull or aching pain, but acute presentations with severe throbbing, sharp pain, or even thunderclap headache may be seen. Anterolateral cervical pain associated with frontal-temporal headache or orbital/facial pain is usually the initial manifestation before ischemic symptoms.[5,6] Similarly, transient ischemic attacks or transient monocular blindness can precede frank cerebral and retinal infarcts, with a relatively short time interval (less than 7 days) in progressing to completed infarction.[6]

Unilateral oculosympathetic palsy compels exclusion of an internal carotid artery dissection even in the absence of other signs or symptoms. The mechanism is related to compression of the third order postganglionic sympathetic fibers ascending along the internal carotid artery or ischemia of the vasa nervosum. The typical manifestations are miosis (constricted pupil) with dilatation lag, ptosis (drooping upper eyelid from loss of sympathetic innervation to the Müller, or superior tarsal muscle), and upside down ptosis (slight elevation of the lower lid). Anhidrosis is specifically not observed due to innervation of the facial sweat glands from the sympathetic plexus of the external carotid artery that is typically excluded from dissections.

Vertebral artery dissections are associated with posterior neck/occipital pain and posterior cerebral or brainstem/cerebellar ischemia. Although occipital neck pain may be easily dismissed for musculoskeletal symptoms, as many as 80% to 90% of patients will eventually develop ischemic sequelae from either flow limiting dissections, or more likely, thromboembolic events.[1,5]

Brainstem/cerebellar ischemia from vertebral artery dissections is most frequently observed in the distribution of the affected posterior inferior cerebellar artery and commonly presents with lateral medullary (Wallenberg) syndrome. Dysfunction of the vestibular system, nucleus ambiguous, inferior cerebellar peduncle, lateral spinothalamic tract, or spinal trigeminal nucleus can result in nystagmus, diplopia, vertigo, nausea and vomiting, unilateral hearing loss, dysphagia, hoarseness, diminished gag reflex, ataxia, dysmetria, dysarthria and sensory deficits of the contralateral body and ipsilateral face. Occipital lobe ischemia in the posterior cerebral artery distributions may lead to bilateral visual deficits.[1,7]

Less common manifestations of vertebral artery dissections include cervical radiculopathy from direct compression of the spinal nerve roots, spinal cord ischemia from compromise of the anterior and posterior spinal arteries or radiculomedullary artery (artery of cervical enlargement), and spinal epidural hematoma from hemorrhagic complications. Approximately 10% of vertebral artery dissections extend intracranially with the potential to rupture or form dissecting aneurysms, thereby presenting with subarachnoid hemorrhage.[1,7]

DIAGNOSTIC IMAGING
Ultrasound

Doppler ultrasound may be used for the initial screening and diagnosis of mid-cervical dissections, but its ability to assess the proximal carotid and vertebral arteries and distal cervical/intracranial vasculature is limited due to interference from the thoracic inlet, mandible, and skull base. Additionally, evaluation of the vertebral arteries is challenging as they course through the foramen tranversarium with specific findings detectable in only 20% of patients.[8]

Although flow pattern abnormalities may be identified because of dissection related stenosis in more than 90% of patients, these are nonspecific findings demonstrating either decreased velocity with high resistance (stenosis), a biphasic pattern (occlusion), or compensatory elevated velocities. More specific findings include segmental dilatation, double lumen with echogenic flap, eccentric echogenic hematoma surrounding a narrowed arterial lumen, and low or absent flow velocity in the dissected false lumen. However, these findings are observed in less than one third of cases and most, if not all, patients will require further noninvasive cross-sectional imaging or conventional angiography.[1,8,9]

Digital Subtraction Angiography

Digital subtraction angiography (DSA) has been considered the gold standard to diagnose or exclude cervical dissections. Along with three-dimensional (3D) rotational DSA techniques, its superior resolution allows the detection of subtle pathognomonic features such as intimal flaps or the double lumen sign, but these are seen in less than 10% of dissections. The most common angiographic finding is a string sign, smooth tapered (or slightly irregular) luminal narrowing in approximately 65% of patients that may progress to an abrupt tapered, flame-like internal carotid artery occlusion (**Fig. 1**A, F). A characteristic location is 2 to 3 cm distal to the carotid bulb with variable extension into the mid or distal cervical segment of the internal carotid artery, though migration is limited by the osseous foramen of the petrous carotid canal. In the vertebral artery, the V1 and V3 segment at the points of entry (C6-C7) and exit (C1-C2 loops) from the foramen transversarium also appear to be common locations for cervical dissections. Location of the pathology and involvement of long segments in cervical dissections assists in differentiation from atherosclerotic disease.[1,9]

Subadventitial dissections result in dissecting aneurysms or pseudoaneurysms in 25% to 35% of patients. The dissecting aneurysms are often fusiform or oval in shape and extend parallel to the arterial lumen. Termed a pearl and string sign, dissecting aneurysms are often seen at the distal margin of a stenotic segment on DSA.[9] Rupture of a mid-cervical dissecting aneurysm may cause the formation of carotid-cutaneous or carotid-pharyngeal fistula with contrast extravasation and arteriovenous shunting best identified on DSA imaging.

Other angiographic findings may include distal thromboembolic branch occlusions of the intracranial arteries that may be difficult to appreciate on cross-sectional imaging. In addition, DSA accurately depicts flow directionality and intracranial transit time, and remains the best modality to assess the collateral intracranial circulation. DSA is superior to cross-sectional imaging studies in evaluating flow-limiting dissections, dissections complicated by arteriovenous fistulas, and flow remodeling after stent placement.

Although DSA is the optimal technique to assess the arterial lumen, its major limitation is its inability to directly image the vessel wall. Therefore, it may be inferior to cross-sectional techniques in the evaluation of nonstenotic dissections with benign intramural hematomas or thrombosed pseudoaneurysms. Another disadvantage of DSA is its potential for ischemic complications. However, the incidence of major neurologic complications from DSA is very low if it is performed by experienced and well-trained physicians.[10] Since multiple vessel dissections occur in up to 25% of patients, careful diagnostic analysis should include bilateral carotid and vertebral artery injections with proximal catheter positioning (proximal common carotid or subclavian arteries) to prevent further injury of a dissected vessel segment and to visualize the entire cervical course and intracranial vasculature.

Computed Tomography Angiography

Noncontrast CT may be useful in evaluating thromboembolic complications of dissections, subacute infarcts, or subarachnoid hemorrhage from intracranial dissections or dissecting aneurysms. CTA is rapidly emerging as a highly sensitive and specific modality for large and medium vessel pathologies of the head and neck.[11] Multi-detector technology enables capture of peak contrast enhancement yielding exceptional detail to evaluate the vessel lumen in addition to the vessel wall. Axial thin-section (0.625 mm–1.25 mm) scanning with enhanced postprocessing capability allows multiplanar reformatted images, 3D reconstructions, and curved maximum intensity projections in virtually any orientation of the vessel (**Fig. 1**B). In a recent study comparing CTA and MRA, Virtinsky and colleagues show CTA to be the preferred cross-sectional modality to delineate the imaging features of cervical dissections, especially for vertebral artery dissections.[12] CTA imaging provides accurate measurements of vessel lumen diameter and dissection length and can provide useful information in treatment planning if endovascular stent reconstruction is planned.

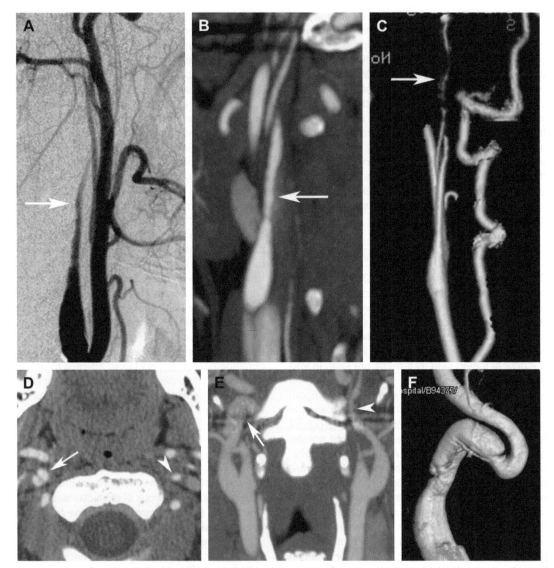

Fig. 1. Imaging of cervical dissections. (*A*) Lateral DSA, (*B*) sagittal reformatted CTA, and (*C*) 3D contrast enhanced (CE) MRA. These images show tapered and slightly irregular narrowing of the right internal carotid artery (*arrows*) just distal to the carotid bulb consistent with a dissection. (*D*) Axial and (*E*) coronal reformatted CTA images in an another patient demonstrate bilateral cervical dissections. The left internal carotid artery demonstrates tapered narrowing (*arrowheads*) along a long segment extending to the skull base, though the periluminal hematoma is not well appreciated. The right internal carotid artery demonstrates an enlarged diameter (*arrows*) with double lumens separated by an intimal flap consistent with a double-barrel dissection, which was confirmed on 3D DSA imaging (*F*).

In the carotid or vertebral arteries, CTA findings of an irregular, narrowed contrast enhancing lumen are indicative of dissection. Vessel wall thickening is often identified on CTA from a subintimal or intramural hematoma and it frequently corresponds with a methemoglobin crescent sign on MRA.[12] A discrete intimal flap or patent double lumens are rarely seen findings (**Fig.** 1D, E). Dissecting aneurysms may be readily identified as focal outpouchings of the enhancing arterial lumen, with or without associated thrombus, and often in an orientation parallel to the vessel.[12]

A relative limitation of CTA imaging is difficulty in its interpretation when extensive calcifications are present along the arterial wall. Furthermore, streak and beam hardening artifact from a patient's dental hardware may limit evaluation of the mid-cervical internal carotid artery, a commonly involved site for dissections. Although recent advances in dynamic CTA with 256 and 320 multi-slice CT scanners may capture both arterial and venous phases, at this time, flow directionality and transit times are best analyzed on DSA.

MR Imaging and MR Angiography

MR imaging and MRA remain the initial screening modality of choice to evaluate patients with suspected cervical dissections. MR imaging with fat saturated axial T1 and T2 weighted sequences provides a sensitive technique to identify subtle dissections where no significant luminal narrowing or mural thickening may be appreciated on DSA or CTA. In fact, the periluminal (subintimal or intramural) hematoma may be uniquely identified on MR imaging in the subacute stage (3–14 days).[9]

The classic finding is circumferential or crescentic hyperintense signal peripheral to the flow void of an irregularly narrowed internal carotid or vertebral artery. Depending on the stage and composition of the hemorrhagic products, the signal on T1 and T2 weighted sequences may vary. In the acute stage (1–3 days), deoxyhemoglobin (T1 isointense and T2 hypointense) may not be apparent and can be difficult to detect. Conversely, methemoglobin in the early subacute stage (3–7 days) causes T1 shortening (T1 hyperintensity) that is easily recognizable against the adjacent flow void. Extracellular methemoglobin in the late subacute stage (7–14+ days) demonstrates T1 and T2 hyperintensity also facilitating detection (Fig 2A, B). Fat suppression techniques are invaluable in differentiating periluminal hematoma from the periarterial fat.[9,13] Recent studies at our institution suggest that presence of restricted diffusion on diffusion weighted imaging (DWI) of the neck may also provide increased sensitivity for detection of intramural hematomas and detection of cervical dissections (Fig. 2C, D) (H. Parmar, unpublished data, 2008). Additionally, since both head and neck imaging are routinely performed, screening for ischemic intracranial complications can be simultaneously performed using DWI.

Other MR imaging findings include the detection of an intimal flap, which may be seen at the proximal end of a dissection, as a thin band of T2 hypointensity separating the residual lumen and periluminal hematoma. However, a distinct intimal flap between double patent lumens is infrequently seen. A highly sensitive and specific finding is an enlarged external diameter of the dissected arterial segment. Occasional contrast enhancement of the intramural hematoma may be appreciated on 3D spoiled gradient-recalled acquisition in the steady state sequence, possibly due to neovascularity, hematoma expansion, or slow residual flow.[9,13]

A 3D contrast-enhanced MRA of the neck offers a sensitive noninvasive technique to assess the cervical vasculature. It has surpassed traditional time of flight (TOF) techniques with higher spatial resolution and elimination of flow artifacts such as in-plane dephasing at arterial bends and signal loss due to slow or turbulent flow in carotid stenosis or pseudoaneurysms. Similar to CTA, post-processing with 3D maximum intensity projections or multiplanar imaging assists in diagnosis of dissections and dissecting aneurysms (Fig. 1C). It is important to remember that subacute periluminal thrombus demonstrates T1 hyperintensity (methemoglobin) on 3D contrast-enhanced or TOF MRA imaging, albeit less intense than flow-related enhancement along the vessel lumen. Therefore, correlation with axial T1 and T2 weighted sequences is recommended in suspected dissections to exclude intramural hematomas, which may not be evident on MRA imaging alone.[9,14]

Although MR imaging exhibits exceptional contrast resolution, spatial and temporal resolution is lower relative to CTA and DSA studies. Increased scanning times are also required in TOF MRA, perhaps explaining a decreased sensitivity for vertebral artery dissections with this technique.[9,12] Phase-contrast MRA and newer dynamic MRA time-resolved techniques allow assessment of flow directionality, velocity, and even transit times to detect flow limiting dissections, but flow patterns are best appreciated qualitatively with DSA at this time.

CT and MR Perfusion

Brain perfusion imaging can demonstrate alterations in cerebral blood flow from proximal cervical dissections. These techniques provide further insight into brain physiology and can assist in therapeutic decision making. In particular, CT perfusion studies provide measurements of cerebral blood flow (CBF), cerebral blood volume (CBV), and mean transit time (MTT) and thereby can quantify the ischemic penumbra. Specifically, decreased CBF (< 40 mL/100 g/min) and elevated MTT (> 6 sec) with preserved cerebral blood volume are observed in noninfarcted, but ischemic or oligemic gray matter.

In the setting of recurrent ischemic symptoms from chronic dissections or asymptomatic progressing dissections, CT perfusion imaging is helpful in the assessment of cerebrovascular reserve. In such patients, there is a need to distinguish tissue that may benefit from increased CBF (tissue under

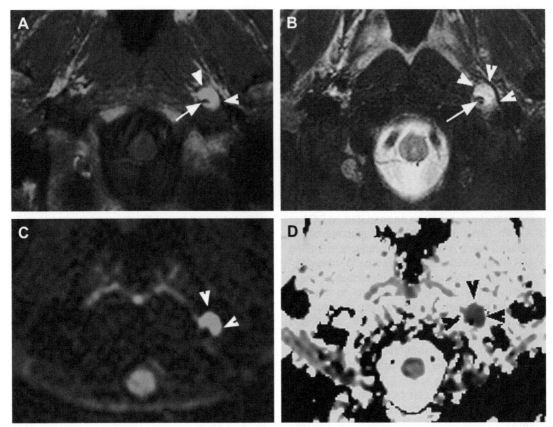

Fig. 2. MR imaging of cervical dissections. (*A*) Axial T1 and (*B*) axial T2 weighted MR images exhibit hyperintense subintimal or intramural hematoma (*arrowheads*) along the left internal carotid artery compatible with a late subacute dissection. Note the flow voids (*arrows*) representing a patent, but narrowed true lumen. (*C*) Axial diffusion weighted image and (*D*) apparent diffusion coefficient mapping demonstrate hyperintense periluminal signal with corresponding low apparent diffusion coefficient values (*arrowheads*) suggestive of restricted diffusion within the intramural hematoma.

hemodynamic stress) from tissue with decreased CBF due to decreased metabolic demand. Cerebrovascular reserve can be evaluated by a tolerance test using intravenous infusion of acetazolamide followed by quantitative CBF measurements. Acetazolamide normally causes vasodilatation of cerebral arterioles and a compensatory increase in CBF. However, patients with hemodynamic ischemic stress are already maximally vasodilated due to the cerebral autoregulatory mechanisms and fail to respond to acetazolamide. These patients are considered to be at increased risk of stroke and may be appropriate candidates to pursue endovascular stent reconstruction.

MEDICAL TREATMENT

Nearly 85% of extracranial dissections and at least 36% of dissecting aneurysms heal spontaneously. It is estimated that greater than 90% of dissection

related infarcts are caused by thromboembolic rather than hemodynamic causes with transcranial Doppler studies confirming passage of microemboli.[15,16] Despite a lack of randomized prospective studies, interval treatment with anticoagulation therapy is advocated to prevent thromboembolic complications.[3,15,17–19]

Anticoagulation therapy with intravenous heparin followed by oral warfarin intake at a target international normalized ratio of 2.0 to 3.0 is the standard treatment for 3 to 6 months. Follow-up MR/MRA imaging is performed at 3 months and 6 months with an expected high rate of dissection healing and recanalization at 3 months (**Fig.** 3A–D). If a dissection-related abnormality persists at 6 months, warfarin treatment is usually discontinued in preference for antiplatelet therapy. The majority of dissecting aneurysms that persist either remain stable or decrease in size with a relatively benign course, hence treatment of dissecting

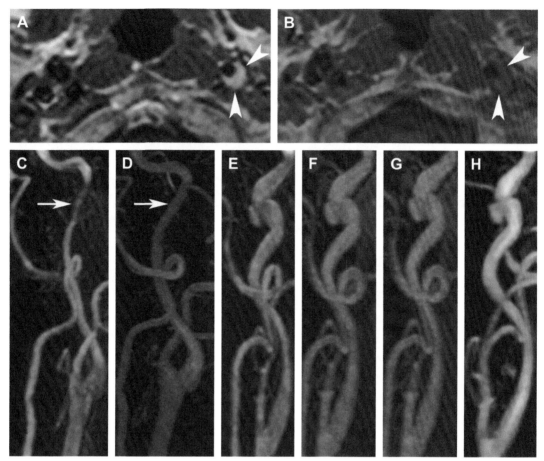

Fig. 3. Medical treatment of cervical dissections and dissecting aneurysms with anticoagulation or antiplatelet therapy. (A) Axial T1 weighted MR image redemonstrates a left internal carotid artery dissection with hyperintense periluminal hematoma (*arrowheads*). Vessel narrowing in the distal cervical segment in this same patient is best seen on 3D CE MRA maximum intensity projection (MIP) (*C, arrow*). (B) Following anticoagulation for 3 months, maturing periluminal hematoma is observed with isointese signal on axial T1-weighted imaging (*arrowheads*). Please also note improved appearance of the vessel caliber on a 3D CE MRA MIP image performed on the same day (*D, arrow*). (E) In another patient treated with anticoagulation and subsequent antiplatelet therapy, dissecting aneurysm (*E*) in the distal cervical segment of the internal carotid artery remains stable at 12 months (*F*), 18 months (*G*) and 30 months (*H*).

aneurysms is not indicated unless they are symptomatic, enlarging, or ruptured (**Fig.** 3E–H).[17–19]

Antiplatelet therapy may be substituted for anticoagulation to avoid iatrogenic hemorrhagic complications in patients with dissections without ischemic symptoms, bleeding diathesis, asymptomatic intracranial dissections, or recent large infarcts. Although aspirin (ASA, or acetylsalicylic acid) is most commonly used at variable doses (325 mg at our institution), no study has directly compared other antiplatelet or anticoagulation agents such as clopidogrel, ticlopidine, or low molecular weight heparin. The recent Cervical Artery Dissection in Stroke Study will examine anticoagulation (heparin or warfarin) versus individual and combined antiplatelet medications in a randomized prospective multicenter trial.[1,3,20]

SURGICAL OR ENDOVASCULAR TREATMENT

Early surgical or endovascular treatment is recommended in symptomatic patients refractory to medical treatment to prevent further thromboembolic complications, or in patients with contraindications to anticoagulation, such as impending infarct, enlarging/ruptured dissecting aneurysm, intracranial dissection/pseudoaneurysm, intracranial or subarachnoid hemorrhage.[3,6]

In some cases, asymptomatic dissections with persisting stenosis, hemodynamic flow limiting

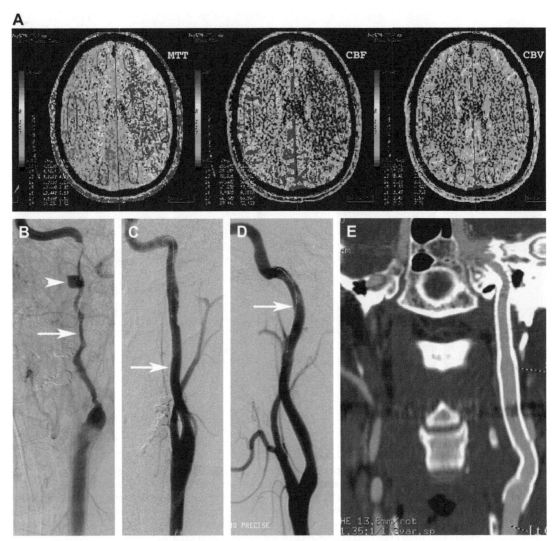

Fig. 4. Endovascular treatment of cervical dissections with self-expanding carotid stent. This patient presented with left hemispheric ischemic symptoms following a left internal carotid artery dissection. (*A*) Brain Perfusion imaging reveals elevated MTT and decreased CBF in the left hemisphere and right anterior cerebral artery territory. The CBV is normal in the corresponding areas. These findings indicate presence of large area of ischemic penumbra (salvageable tissue without infarction). (*B*) Anteroposterior oblique DSA images demonstrate a flow limiting progressing dissection involving nearly the entire cervical course of the left internal carotid artery. Severe irregular narrowing along the cervical segment (arrow) is also associated with an eccentric contrast saccule (arrowhead) suggestive of a small dissecting aneurysm. (*C–D, arrows*) Endovascular treatment with sequential placement of tandem self-expanding carotid stents reconstructs the left internal carotid artery securing the intimal flap and re-constituting flow in the expanded vessel lumen. Note decreased opacification of the pseudoaneurysm presumably due to realignment of the intimal flap or flow remodeling. (*E*) On follow-up, coronal reformatted CTA image delineates dissection healing and successful stent reconstruction of the cervical left internal carotid artery with no residual stenosis or pseudoaneurysm. (*Courtesy of* Nasser Razack, MD, Saint Petersburg, FL.)

stenosis, or unstable intimal flaps may also be aggressively treated,[17,21] though there are no established criteria to treat these lesions before the failure of medical management. Since the incidence of thromboembolic complications from persistent stenosis or nonhealing dissections is approximately doubled (0.7% versus 0.3%), an argument can be made to treat these lesions.[17] Some have supported treatment based upon analogous data from the carotid atherosclerosis trials that demonstrated the benefits of carotid endarterectomy over medical management in symptomatic patients with greater than 50% to 70% carotid stenosis,[22,23] asymptomatic patients with greater than 60% carotid stenosis,[10] and carotid stenting over endarterectomy in high risk patients with symptomatic severe carotid stenosis.[24]

Cervical dissections may be treated with surgical ligation to deconstruct the carotid or vertebral arteries with or without extracranial to intracranial bypass techniques. However, high complication rates of ischemic injury or cranial nerve deficits, specifically the pharyngeal and superior laryngeal branches of the vagus nerve, have been reported due to technically demanding skull base exposure. Furthermore, most dissecting aneurysms are fusiform and rarely amenable to surgical clipping with vessel reconstruction.[3,25,26]

Although simple vessel deconstruction may also be performed with endovascular coils, Amplatzer plug (AGA Medical, Plymouth, MN) or detachable balloon occlusion, the risk of delayed ischemia caused by thrombus propagation, emboli, or hemodynamic insufficiency is similar to surgical ligation. An endovascular balloon test occlusion study is recommended to assess the patient's collateral circulation and cerebrovascular reserve (or requirement for bypass) to prevent a hemodynamic infarct after vessel sacrifice. Despite successful balloon occlusion testing, a small risk of infarction remains, and therefore, preservation of intracranial blood flow is the preferable alternative.[27]

Endovascular stent reconstruction is the primary interventional option over endovascular/surgical vessel deconstruction or surgical bypass. It is an effective and relatively safe technique, but studies have been limited to multiple case reports and retrospective small case series involving both the carotid and vertebral arteries.[28–36] Because of the low incidence of carotid dissections, even the largest series reported by Kadkhodayan and colleagues[21] consisted of only 26 subjects that were treated with stent placement or stent angioplasty.

The technique involves placement of a 6 French guide sheath or 8 French guide catheter proximal to the level of dissection in the common carotid or subclavian-vertebral arteries. Dedicated cervical and intracranial angiograms assist in pre-treatment planning. Specifically, the degree of dissection related stenosis, arterial diameter measurements and length of the injured vessel segment are precisely calculated. Additionally, the presence of flow-limitation, mural thrombus, dissecting aneurysm, and the baseline intracranial vasculature can be evaluated. Through the guide sheath or catheter, a microwire-microcatheter complex is carefully advanced across the narrowed arterial segment utilizing fluoroscopic roadmap guidance. It is imperative to advance across the dissection cautiously, remaining within the true vessel lumen. Intermittent proximal check angiograms or microcatheter angiograms with gentle contrast hand injections are used to confirm access through the true lumen, opacifying the normal distal vessel and intracranial vasculature. Utilized in peripheral interventions, intravascular ultrasound may have a future role in directing intraluminal wire placement.

Distal filter protection devices are not warranted in the treatment of cervical dissections, unlike atherosclerotic lesions which have a greater potential for thromboemboli during carotid angioplasty and stent deployment. In addition, if used in the treatment of dissections, there is a risk of further intimal injury or dissection progression during advancement and deployment of these relatively rigid filter devices. Pre- and post-stent balloon angioplasty has been reported in the endovascular treatment of internal carotid artery dissections.[21,29,30,33] However, the indications for angioplasty in the treatment of dissections are very limited, usually to obtain access across the stenosis or salvage an incompletely expanded stent. In rare cases, angioplasty alone has been shown to achieve sufficient luminal expansion in symptomatic vertebral-basilar artery dissections.[34,35]

Following selection of a stent based on sizing criteria, vessel tortuosity, and specific stent characteristics (flexibility, radial force, metal-mesh ratio, deployment mechanism), it is advanced across the dissection flap or dissecting aneurysm and deployed using rapid exchange or over-the-wire techniques. Final cervical and intracranial angiograms assess post-stent reconstruction of the vessel wall: adequacy of luminal expansion, uniform stent apposition to the vessel wall, improvement in flow dynamics, in-stent thrombus formation, or distal intracranial thromboembolic complications.

Stent placement expands the true lumen of a dissected vessel to reestablish blood flow, realign the intimal flap, and trap the subintimal hematoma. Over the next several weeks to months, hematoma resorption, intimal healing, and stent endothelialization reconstructs the parent artery. Furthermore, flow remodeling through the stent may promote pseudoaneurysm thrombosis secondary to intimal apposition, reduced porosity through the stent mesh (decreased intra-aneurysmal inflow velocity and vorticity), and eventual stent endothelialization based on aneurysm flow models and animal experiments.[37,38] Alternatively, the stent provides scaffolding for pseudoaneurysm treatment with coil embolization to protect the parent artery.

Endovascular treatment of simple carotid dissections is predominantly performed with porous self-expanding carotid stents, which are more flexible and easier to advance into the cervical vasculature.[21,28–33,36] In the smaller vertebral arteries, lower profile balloon-expanding coronary stents may be required.

Balloon-expanding coronary stents possess advantageous properties in the treatment of cervical dissections generally with greater radial force and metal-mesh ratio than self-expanding stents. Stent functionality is proportional to circumferential force which maintains patency of the dissected artery, expanding the true lumen and tacking up the intimal flap. The higher metal-mesh ratio decreases the porosity across the inflow zone to allow intimal healing and may secure preexisting thrombus along the dissected vessel wall, preventing intracranial migration. Both radial force and metal matrix have been postulated to indirectly augment flow remodeling by triggering an intimal response and stent endothelialization; thereby promoting intra-aneurysmal thrombosis or parent artery reconstruction.[37–39]

Interestingly, several case reports have shown the spontaneous thrombosis of dissecting carotid and vertebral artery aneurysms after placement of overlapping balloon-expanding stents using the double stent or stent-within-a stent technique,[40–42] presumably due to the combined radial force against the intimal flap and decreased porosity through the interstices of two stents. In fact, spontaneous healing of a few dissecting fusiform and even true saccular/fusiform intracranial aneurysms have been reported using a single balloon-expanding stent.[43–45]

Conversely, balloon-expanding stents are relatively inflexible and difficult to advance across tortuous or redundant vessel segments. Although somewhat improved with newer delivery systems, balloon-expanding stents are inherently noncompliant and can exert excessive radial force during deployment in dissected or fragile distal cervical/intracranial vasculature leading to vessel dissection or rupture. Using these rigid stents at the craniocervical junction and skull base may lead to crimping of the stent or kinking of the parent vessel during neck flexion or extension with grave consequences.

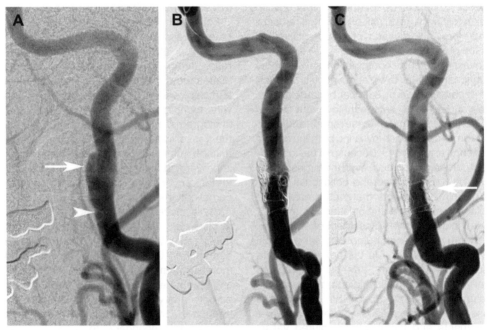

Fig. 5. Endovascular treatment of cervical dissection and dissecting aneurysm with stent reconstruction and coil embolization. This 51-year-old woman status post neck trauma presented with neck pain and episodes of left hemispheric transient ischemic attacks. (*A*) AP DSA image shows a left internal carotid artery dissection (*arrowhead*). Additionally, longitudinal irregularity with a medially projecting broad based dissecting aneurysm is seen (*arrow*). (*B*) Following self-expanding carotid stent placement and coil embolization of the dissecting aneurysm, the intimal flap is apposed to the vessel wall with improved true lumen diameter and near complete thrombosis of the dissecting aneurysm (*arrow*). (*C*) On 1-year follow-up, complete healing with further thrombosis of the dissecting aneurysm has occurred secondary to coil embolization and stent-induced flow remodeling (*arrow*).

Furthermore, the greater metal matrix of balloon-expanding stents may predispose to increased foreign body reaction and platelet aggregation resulting in thromboembolic complications or myointimal proliferation, especially in the setting of preexisting endothelial injury.[37]

Self-expanding carotid stents are designed for atraumatic deployment with decreased, yet adequate, radial force to treat atherosclerotic lesions. Successful treatment of internal carotid artery dissections with these stents has been extensively described (**Figs. 4** and **5**).[21,28–33,36] Atypical for most self-expanding stents, newer carotid stents have been designed with both enhanced radial force (nitinol stents, eg, Precise stent, Cordis, Miami Lakes, FL) and greater metal matrix (closed cell designs, eg, Wallstent). Such self-expanding, closed cell carotid stents include the X-Act (Abbott Vascular Devices, Galway, Ireland) or NexStent (Boston Scientific, Natick, MA) systems and may provide equally effective and safer alternatives to balloon-expanding stents in proximal to mid-cervical dissections and dissecting aneurysms.

Although new 5F carotid delivery systems are promising, the high profile and rigid construction of self-expanding carotid stents prevents their routine use in the distal internal carotid and vertebral arteries. Furthermore, the trackability of both self-expanding carotid stents and balloon-expanding coronary stents is limited in tortuous anatomy, redundant vessels, or high cervical/skull base segments. In these situations, self-expanding dedicated intracranial stents are quite useful due to their inherent low profile and flexible properties. Intracranial stents can provide adequate radial force and atraumatic expansion in treating distal dissections.[46,47]

Covered stent grafts have been used in the simultaneous treatment of dissections and dissecting aneurysms (**Fig. 6**) and are convenient devices in excluding giant pseudoaneurysms or carotid cavernous fistulas resulting from a ruptured pseudoaneurysm.[30,33,48–53] Adverse properties include high-profile delivery systems, limited trackability in tortuous vasculature, occlusion risk to perforating arteries, and lack of long term patency data. Though self-expanding covered stent grafts are now available, the reported literature favors uncovered balloon or self-expanding stents for the treatment of arterial dissections

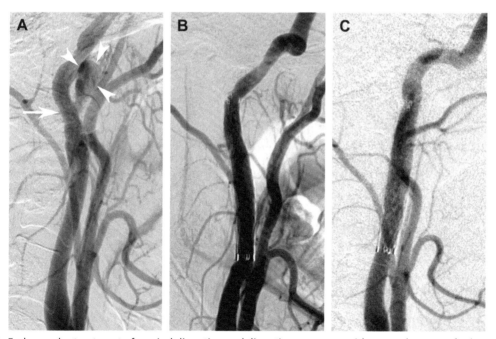

Fig. 6. Endovascular treatment of cervical dissection and dissecting aneurysm with covered stent graft placement. A 19-year-old woman presents status post motor-vehicle accident with persistent right-sided headache and pulsatile tinnitus (*A*) Lateral DSA image demonstrates segmental vessel narrowing in the distal cervical right internal carotid artery (*arrow*) indicative of dissection. A saccular appearing pseudoaneurysm (*arrowheads*) arises anteriorly and superiorly from this narrowed segment. (*B*) Following self-expanding covered stent graft placement, there is resulting normal vessel diameter and exclusion of the pseudoaneurysm with no residual opacification. (*C*) On 6-month follow-up, complete healing of the right internal carotid artery has occurred with no residual dissection-related stenosis or aneurysm opacification.

with subsequent coil embolization through the stent interstices to manage dissecting aneurysms (see **Fig. 5**).[21,28,30,31,36,46]

Thromboembolic complications and intimal hyperplasia causing hemodynamically significant in-stent stenosis are well documented following metallic stent placement in the cervical and intracranial vasculature. The prevention of acute thromboembolic complications entails the routine use of systemic heparin (activated clotting time 2.0–2.5 times baseline) during endovascular procedures. The inherent thrombogenicity of metallic stents mandates antiplatelet therapy as a pre- and postprocedure supplement to heparinization in such cases. Our standard protocol is an antiplatelet regimen (75 mg clopidogrel and 81 mg ASA daily) for 5 days or a loading bolus (300 mg clopidogrel and 650 mg ASA) 1 day before stent placement and dual antiplatelet therapy (75 mg clopidogrel and 81 mg ASA daily) after stent placement for at least 12 weeks. In emergent situations, a loading bolus of 400 to 600 mg clopidogel approximately 2 to 5 hours before an endovascular procedure also achieves maximum platelet inhibition.[54] Routine Doppler ultrasound and clinical follow-up is recommended at 3-month intervals for 1 year to detect complications of intimal hyperplasia, in-stent stenosis, or thrombosis.

REFERENCES

1. Schievink WI. Spontaneous dissection of the carotid and vertebral arteries. N Engl J Med 2001;344(12): 898–906.
2. Brandt T, Orberk E, Weber R, et al. Pathogenesis of cervical artery dissections: association with connective tissue abnormalities. Neurology 2001;57(1): 24–30.
3. Schievink WI. The treatment of spontaneous carotid and vertebral artery dissections. Curr Opin Cardiol 2000;15(5):316–21.
4. Hufnagel A, Hammers A, Schönle PW, et al. Stroke following chiropractic manipulation of the cervical spine. J Neurol 1999;246(8):683–8.
5. Silbert PL, Mokri B, Shievink WI. Headache and neck pain in spontaneous internal carotid and vertebral artery dissections. Neurology 1995;45(8):1517–22.
6. Biousse V, D'Anglejan-Chatillon J, Touboul PJ, et al. Time course of symptoms in extracranial carotid artery dissections. A series of 80 patients. Stroke 1995;26(2):235–9.
7. Caplan LR, Zarins CK, Hemmati M. Spontaneous dissection of the extracranial vertebral arteries. Stroke 1985;16(6):1030–8.
8. Gardner DJ, Gosink BB, Kallman CE. Internal carotid artery dissections: duplex ultrasound imaging. J Ultrasound Med 1991;10(11):607–14.
9. Provenzale JM. Dissection of the internal carotid and vertebral arteries: imaging features. AJR Am J Roentgenol 1995;165(5):1099–104.
10. Endarterectomy for asymptomatic carotid artery stenosis. Executive Committee for the Asymptomatic Carotid Atherosclerosis Study. JAMA 1995; 273(18):1421–8.
11. Villablanca JP, Rodriguez FJ, Stockman T, et al. MDCT angiography for detection and quantification of small intracranial arteries: comparison with conventional catheter angiography. AJR Am J Roentgenol 2007;188(2):593–602.
12. Vertinsky AT, Schwartz NE, Fischbein NJ, et al. Comparison of multidetector CT angiography and MR imaging of cervical artery dissection. AJNR Am J Neuroradiol 2008;29(9):1753–60.
13. Bousson V, Lévy C, Brunereau L, et al. Dissections of the internal carotid artery: three-dimensional time-of-flight MR angiography and MR imaging features. AJR Am J Roentgenol 1999;173(1):139–43.
14. Phan T, Huston J 3rd, Bernstein MA, et al. Contrast-enhanced magnetic resonance angiography of the cervical vessels: experience with 422 patients. Stroke 2001;32(10):2282–6.
15. Lucas C, Moulin T, Deplanque D, et al. Stroke patterns of internal carotid artery dissection in 40 patients. Stroke 1998;29(12):2646–8.
16. Srinivasan J, Newell DW, Sturzenegger M, et al. Transcranial Doppler in the evaluation of internal carotid artery dissection. Stroke 1996;27(7): 1226–30.
17. Kremer C, Mosso M, Georgiadis D, et al. Carotid dissection with permanent and transient occlusion or severe stenosis: long-term outcome. Neurology 2003;60(2):271–5.
18. Mokri B, Sundt TM Jr, Houser OW, et al. Spontaneous dissection of the cervical internal carotid artery. Ann Neurol 1986;19(2):126–38.
19. Touze E, Randoux B, Meary E, et al. Aneurysmal forms of cervical artery dissection: associated factors and outcome. Stroke 2001;32(2):418–23.
20. Cervical Artery Dissection in Stroke Study Trial Investigators. Antiplatelet therapy vs. anticoagulation in cervical artery dissection: rationale and design of the Cervical Artery Dissection in Stroke Study (CADISS). Int J Stroke 2007;2(4):292–6.
21. Kadkhodayan Y, Jeck DT, Moran CJ, et al. Angioplasty and stenting in carotid dissection with or without associated pseudoaneurysm. AJNR Am J Neuroradiol 2005;26(9):2328–35.
22. North American Symptomatic Carotid Endarterectomy Trial Collaborators. Beneficial effect of carotid endarterectomy in symptomatic patients with high-grade stenosis. N Engl J Med 1991;325:445–53.
23. Barnett HJ, Taylor DW, Eliasziw M, et al. Benefit of carotid endarterectomy in patients with symptomatic moderate or severe stenosis. North American

Symptomatic Carotid Endarterectomy Trial Collaborators. N Engl J Med 1998;339(20):1415–25.

24. Yadav JS, Wholey MH, Kuntz RE, et al.Stenting and Angioplasty with Protection in Patients at High Risk for Endarterectomy Investigators. Protected carotid-artery stenting versus endarterectomy in high-risk patients. N Engl J Med 2004;351(15):1493–501.

25. Muller BT, Luther B, Hort W, et al. Surgical treatment of 50 carotid dissections: indications and results. J Vasc Surg 2000;31(5):980–8.

26. Schievink WI, Piepgras DG, McCaffrey TV, et al. Surgical treatment of extracranial internal carotid artery dissecting aneurysms. Neurosurgery 1994; 35(5):809–15.

27. van Rooij WJ, Sluzewski M, Slob MJ, et al. Predictive value of angiographic testing for tolerance to therapeutic occlusion of the carotid artery. AJNR Am J Neuroradiol 2005;26(1):175–8.

28. Malek AM, Higashida RT, Phatouros CC, et al. Endovascular management of extracranial carotid artery dissection achieved using stent angioplasty. AJNR Am J Neuroradiol 2000;21(7):1280–92.

29. Bejjani GK, Monsein LH, Laird JR, et al. Treatment of symptomatic cervical carotid dissections with endovascular stents. Neurosurgery 1999;44(4):755–60.

30. Liu AY, Paulsen RD, Marcellus ML, et al. Long-term outcomes after carotid stent placement treatment of carotid artery dissection. Neurosurgery 1999; 45(6):1368–73.

31. Bush RL, Lin PH, Dodson TF, et al. Endoluminal stent placement and coil embolization for the management of carotid artery pseudoaneurysms. J Endovasc Ther 2001;8(1):53–61.

32. Cohen JE, Ben-Hur T, Rajz G, et al. Endovascular stent-assisted angioplasty in the management of traumatic internal carotid artery dissections. Stroke 2005;36(4):e45–7.

33. Edgell RC, Abou-Chebl A, Yadav JS. Endovascular management of spontaneous carotid artery dissection. J Vasc Surg 2005;42(5):854–60.

34. Willing SJ, Skidmore F, Donaldson J, et al. Treatment of acute intracranial vertebrobasilar dissection with angioplasty and stent placement: report of two cases. AJNR Am J Neuroradiol 2003;24(5):985–9.

35. Cohen JE, Gomori JM, Umansky F. Endovascular management of symptomatic vertebral artery dissection achieved using stent angioplasty and emboli protection device. Neurol Res 2003;25(4):418–22.

36. Ahn JY, Chung SS, Lee BH, et al. Treatment of spontaneous arterial dissections with stent placement for preservation of the parent artery. Acta Neurochir (Wien) 2005;147(3):265–73.

37. Wakhloo AK, Schellhammer F, de Vries J, et al. Self-expanding and balloon-expandable stents in the treatment of carotid aneurysms: an experimental study in a canine model. AJNR Am J Neuroradiol 1994;15(3):493–502.

38. Lieber BB, Stancampiano AP, Wakhloo AK. Alteration of hemodynamics in aneurysm models by stenting: influence of stent porosity. Ann Biomed Eng 1997;25(3):460–9.

39. Fiorella D, Albuquerque FC, Deshmukh VR, et al. Usefulness of the Neuroform stent for the treatment of cerebral aneurysms: results at initial (3-6-mo) follow-up. Neurosurgery 2005;56(6):1191–201.

40. Benndorf G, Herbon U, Sollmann WP, et al. Treatment of a ruptured dissecting vertebral artery aneurysm with double stent placement: case report. AJNR Am J Neuroradiol 2001;22(10):1844–8.

41. Mehta B, Burke T, Kole M, et al. Stent-within-a-stent technique for the treatment of dissecting vertebral artery aneurysms. AJNR Am J Neuroradiol 2003; 24(9):1814–8.

42. Doerfler A, Wanke I, Egelhof T, et al. Double-stent method: therapeutic alternative for small wide-necked aneurysms. Technical note. J Neurosurg 2004;100(1):150–4.

43. Brassel F, Rademaker J, Haupt C, et al. Intravascular stent placement for a fusiform aneurysm of the posterior cerebral artery: case report. Eur Radiol 2001;11(7):1250–3.

44. Lylyk P, Cohen JE, Ceratto R, et al. Endovascular reconstruction of intracranial arteries by stent placement and combined techniques. J Neurosurg 2002; 97(6):1306–13.

45. Vanninen R, Manninen H, Ronkainen A. Broad-based intracranial aneurysms: thrombosis induced by stent placement. AJNR Am J Neuroradiol 2003; 24(2):263–6.

46. Pride GL Jr, Replogle RE, Rappard G, et al. Stent-coil treatment of a distal internal carotid artery dissecting pseudoaneurysm on a redundant loop by use of a flexible, dedicated nitinol intracranial stent. AJNR Am J Neuroradiol 2004;25(2):333–7.

47. Ansari SA, Thompson BG, Gemmete JJ, et al. Endovascular treatment of distal cervical and intracranial dissections with the neuroform stent. Neurosurgery 2008;62(3):636–46.

48. Scavee V, De Wispelaere JF, Mormont E, et al. Pseudoaneurysm of the internal carotid artery: treatment with a covered stent. Cardiovasc Intervent Radiol 2001;24(4):283–5.

49. Tseng A, Ramaiah V, Rodriguez-Lopez JA, et al. Emergent endovascular treatment of a spontaneous internal carotid artery dissection with pseudoaneurysm. J Endovasc Ther 2003;10(3):643–6.

50. Saket RR, Razavi MK, Sze DY, et al. Stent-graft treatment of extracranial carotid and vertebral arterial lesions. J Vasc Interv Radiol 2004;15(10): 1151–6.

51. Heye S, Maleux G, Vandenberghe R, et al. Symptomatic internal carotid artery dissecting pseudoaneurysm: endovascular treatment by stent-graft. Cardiovasc Intervent Radiol 2005;28(4):499–501.

52. Assadian A, Senekowitsch C, Rotter R, et al. Long-term results of covered stent repair of internal carotid artery dissections. J Vasc Surg 2004;40(3):484–7.

53. Felber S, Henkes H, Weber W, et al. Treatment of extracranial and intracranial aneurysms and arterio-venous fistulae using stent grafts. Neurosurgery 2004;55(3):631–8.

54. von Beckerath N, Taubert D, Pogatsa-Murray G, et al. Absorption, metabolization, and antiplatelet effects of 300-, 600-, and 900-mg loading doses of clopidogrel: results of the ISAR-CHOICE (Intracoronary Stenting and Antithrombotic Regimen: Choose Between 3 High Oral Doses for Immediate Clopidogrel Effect) Trial. Circulation 2005;112(19):2946–50.

Update on Endovascular Management of the Carotid Blowout Syndrome

Avi Mazumdar, MD[a,b,c], Colin P. Derdeyn, MD[a,c,d],*,
William Holloway, MD[a], Christopher J. Moran, MD[a,d],
DeWitte T. Cross, III, MD[a,d]

KEYWORDS

- Carotid blowout • Stroke • Endovascular • Hemorrhage
- Stenting • Sacrifice

Carotid blowout syndrome can be a life-threatening late complication of surgical and radiation therapy for head and neck tumors in the vicinity of the cervical carotid artery. The syndrome spans a spectrum of pathology from impending to acute rupture of the artery. These cases are uncommon, can be dramatic in terms of blood loss, and are often true emergencies. The optimal management of these patients requires quick recognition, and often advanced trauma life-support skills and creative endovascular solutions. Definitive endovascular treatment is the therapy of choice in this condition; open surgical options are very limited. In this article, we present some background information regarding the clinical and pathologic aspects of the syndrome and our experience in endovascular management.

HEAD AND NECK TUMOR OVERVIEW

More than 500,000 patients worldwide are diagnosed with squamous cell carcinoma of the head and neck each year. The primary site of the tumor can affect the nasopharynx, oropharynx, larynx, and hypopharynx. Smoking, alcohol abuse, and smokeless tobacco are major risk factors for the development of squamous cell cancer of the head and neck. There are also associations between marijuana use and occupational exposures including nickel refining.

There is increasing evidence to suggest that certain viruses are associated with head and neck tumors. Specifically, human papilloma virus (HPV) has an association with squamous cell cancer of the head and neck. Epstein Barr Virus (EBV) has a specific association with nasopharyngeal cancer. Most head and neck tumors occur in men older than 50 years of age. Presenting symptoms can include sore throat, dysphagia, and odynophagia. Nasopharyngeal cancer can present with sore throat, sinusitis, hoarseness, nasal obstruction, epistaxis, and serous otitis media. Patients with more advanced disease may present with cranial neuropathies or cervical lymphadenopathy.[1]

The TNM (Tumor, Node, Metastases) staging system is used, as for most cancer types. Overall outcomes are better in patients with low-grade disease, with an 80% cure rate in patients with stage I disease, and 60% cure rate in patients with stage II disease. Advanced disease (stage III and Stage IV) has a less than 30% cure rate. Nasopharyngeal cancer in particular will often present

[a] Mallinckrodt Institute of Radiology, Washington University School of Medicine, 510 South Kingshighway Boulevard, St. Louis, MO 63110-1093, USA
[b] Department of Interventional Neuroradiology, Central DuPage Hospital, 3rd Floor Ambulatory Services Pavilion, 25 North Winfield Road, Winfield, IL 60190, USA
[c] Department of Neurology, Washington University School of Medicine, St. Louis, MO, USA
[d] Department of Neurological Surgery, Washington University School of Medicine, St. Louis, MO, USA
* Corresponding author. Washington University School of Medicine, 510 South Kingshighway Boulevard, St. Louis, MO 63110-1093.
E-mail address: derdeync@mir.wustl.edu (C.P. Derdeyn).

Neuroimag Clin N Am 19 (2009) 271–281
doi:10.1016/j.nic.2009.01.001

with nodal metastases, and has a high rate of treatment failure. Organ preservation strategies are preferred when possible. Chemotherapy and radiation therapy are common adjuncts to surgery.[1]

Surgical approaches to patients with head and neck tumors include radical neck dissection, modified radical neck dissection, and selective lymph node dissection.

Radical Neck Dissection

Radical neck dissection involves en bloc removal of the lymph node–bearing tissues on one side of the neck, as well as the removal of the spinal accessory nerve, internal jugular vein (IJV), and sternocleidomastoid muscle. Usually radical lymph node dissections are performed when there are multiple cervical lymph node metastases, particularly involving the posterior triangle of the neck, or if tightly related to the spinal accessory nerve. The presence of a large metastatic tumor mass or matted lymph nodes in the upper part of the neck is also an indication for a radical lymph node dissection. At many institutions, fewer than 20% of neck dissections for tumor are radical lymph node dissections.[2]

Modified Radical Neck Dissection

Modified radical neck dissection attempts to preserve the IJV, the sternocleidomastoid muscle, or the spinal accessory nerve, with the goal of reducing morbidity. Resection of the spinal accessory nerve results in shoulder disability and a cosmetic deformity, which can be avoided sometimes by a modified radical neck dissection.[2]

Selective Lymph Node Dissection

Selective lymph node dissection involves removal of only the lymph node groups at the highest risk of containing metastases.[2]

Radical neck dissection for treatment of primary head and neck tumors can be complicated by carotid artery injury, wound breakdown, and tumor recurrence. Carotid artery rupture occurs primarily if there is thrombosis of the vasa vasorum, which can occur with radiation therapy or surgical stripping of the carotid sheath and has been associated with up to 4% of radical neck dissections.[1,3,4]

CAROTID BLOWOUT SYNDROME

Carotid blowout syndrome is classically defined as rupture of the extracranial carotid artery or its branches. This is usually a result of wound breakdown after surgical and radiation therapy for head and neck cancer or as a result of trauma. This rupture can result in active bleeding into the airway, pseudoaneurysm, or arteriovenous fistula (AVF) formation. Carotid blowout syndrome is associated with high morbidity and mortality, although outcomes have improved with the advent of endovascular treatment modalities.

Radiation therapy, more extensive surgery, wound breakdown, infection, and tumor recurrence are all predisposing factors for the carotid blowout syndrome. Radiation therapy almost certainly weakens the arterial wall, likely by obliterating the vasa vasorum, resulting in an increased risk of carotid blowout syndrome. Although usually seen in patients with major head and neck resections and concurrent radiation therapy, it can also occur in patients who have had radiation therapy only.[5] Patients with radical neck dissections and wound breakdown are at a high risk of carotid artery rupture.[4] Carotid peel, when tumor encasing the carotid artery is surgically removed, also increases chances of a later carotid blowout.

Tumor recurrence is also a predisposing factor for carotid blowout syndrome, especially when the tumor recurrence invades the carotid artery. Wound breakdown from a previous radical neck dissection or flap mobilization can result in an exposed carotid artery. Patients with squamous cell cancer have many factors that contribute to poor wound healing, which can include poor tissue oxygenation, infection, and the long-term presence of mobile foreign bodies (tracheostomy and nasogastric tube placement). Direct exposure to saliva can result in digestion of the vessel wall by salivary enzymes, as occurs in a pharyngocutaneous fistula.

The initial clinical description of carotid blowout syndrome was by Borsany[6] and the first clinical series reported by Ketcham and Hoye.[7] Chaloupka and colleagues[8,9] defined carotid blowout as a syndrome with the following three primary subtypes.

Exposed Carotid Artery

Postoperative wound breakdown from radical neck dissection or flap mobilization can result in an exposed carotid artery. This can be treated with placement of healthy well-vascularized tissue over the exposed carotid artery, or if it is not possible to cover the exposed carotid artery with healthy well-vascularized tissue, with a test balloon occlusion and possible carotid sacrifice. Recently this definition has been expanded to include cases where there is radiologic evidence of tumor extension and neoplastic invasion of the carotid system as well as a nonhemorrhagic pseudoaneurysm on angiography.[10,11]

Impending Carotid Rupture

This subtype refers to patients who present with a sentinel hemorrhage, usually from a pseudoaneurysm. The bleeding in these cases is profuse but self-limited, and can be transoral, transcervical, or through a surgical wound or fistula. An impending carotid rupture is usually from a pseudoaneurysm that leaks intermittently. This type of lesion must be treated emergently.

Acute Carotid Blowout

This subtype refers to acute uncontrolled hemorrhage, which is not controlled with surgical packing. Standard ICU care for these types of patients includes hemodynamic stabilization and airway protection. Adequate venous access is necessary for administration of fluids and blood products, and to maintain an adequate blood pressure. These patients must be treated emergently. Hypotension is a major risk factor for the development of stroke in these patients.

DIAGNOSTIC IMAGING

The affected artery in carotid blowout syndrome can include the common carotid artery, the internal carotid artery, and the external carotid artery or its branches.[9] Vascular imaging tests, in particular CT angiography, are valuable in planning appropriate treatment for these lesions by accurately determining the location of the lesion and guiding therapy. This is true even in the setting of active hemorrhage.

CT Angiography

Computed tomography angiography (CTA) can be a very effective screening examination to evaluate for the site of active extravasation and to identify the underlying vascular lesion, such as a pseudoaneurysm. There is value to this information even in the setting of acute hemorrhage, as the localization of a bleeding source can help target the endovascular procedure and save critical time (Fig. 1). In addition, the images also provide very complementary information to the catheter angiogram regarding the soft tissue (if any!) surrounding the artery (Fig. 2). This can be useful in determining whether to sacrifice the vessel or pursue another vessel-preserving strategy such as a stent. The advantages of CT angiography include its speed, allowing the rapid acquisition of data in an unstable patient, and ready availability in the emergency department and inpatient setting. With high-resolution modern multidetector scanners and advanced postprocessing techniques such as multiplanar reconstruction, an effective roadmap

for further angiographic evaluation and endovascular treatment can be obtained. Disadvantages of using CT angiography as a screening tool include extra contrast administration and additional radiation exposure, which are usually not prominent concerns in this patient population.

Diagnostic Angiography

Diagnostic angiography remains the gold standard for evaluation of patients with carotid blowout syndrome and it allows for endovascular treatment at the time of the procedure. The diagnostic angiogram can be done with anesthesia or with conscious sedation depending on the stability of the patient and his or her mental status. Conventional angiography allows evaluation of the circle of Willis for sources of collateral flow if vessel sacrifice is a potential treatment option. As with CT angiography, identifying the site or source of bleeding allows for targeted intervention.

Important considerations when evaluating an angiogram in a patient with suspected carotid blowout syndrome includes looking for sites of endoluminal irregularity and pseudoaneurysms, as well as for sites of active extravasation. The common carotid artery (CCA), the internal carotid artery (ICA), and the external carotid artery (ECA) must be carefully evaluated. If angiography of these vessels does not reveal a bleeding source, the thyrocervical trunks, costocervical trunks, and subclavian arteries should be evaluated if the bleeding is in the lower part of the neck.[8,9]

TEMPORARY BALLOON OCCLUSION

Abrupt occlusion of the internal carotid artery can result in a stroke in up to 50% of cases.[12,13] In patients who are stable and in whom internal carotid artery occlusion is considered a treatment option, a temporary balloon occlusion test should be performed (Fig. 3). In general, patients with an acute carotid blowout or sentinel hemorrhage will be too unstable to tolerate a balloon occlusion test and should be treated on a more emergent basis. Patients who have an exposed carotid artery, radiographic evidence of invasion of the carotid artery, or a pseudoaneurysm that has not bled should undergo temporary balloon occlusion testing before carotid sacrifice.

Clinical failure rates of permanent balloon occlusion after temporary balloon occlusion are 5% to 20%.[14,15] Some authors have found that this rate can be reduced significantly (3% to 12%) with imaging adjuncts such as technetium-99m (99mTc) hexamethylpropyleneamine oxime (HMPAO) single photon emission computed tomography (SPECT) or Xenon CT.[16,17]

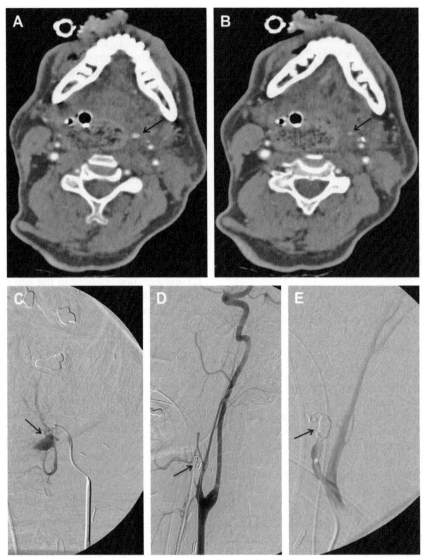

Fig. 1. The patient is a 54-year-old male status post resection of a left tonsillar squamous cell cancer, who presented with profuse uncontrolled oral hemorrhage. The patient had a CTA (*A*), which shows a pseudoaneurysm (*black arrow*) of the left lingual artery. One slice below (*B*) shows the normal caliber of the lingual artery (*black arrow*). Conventional angiography (*C*) with a selective microcatheter injection shows a pseudoaneurysm (*black arrow*) of the lingual artery, which was treated with coil embolization of the pseudoaneurysm. (*D*) Follow-up left common carotid artery injection after coil embolization shows complete exclusion of the pseudoaneurysm (*black arrow*). The remainder of the external carotid artery was then sacrificed (*E*) with coil embolization (*black arrow*). The procedure was performed under conditions of active extravasation, and hypotension despite ongoing resuscitation efforts. Blood pressure improved dramatically after occlusion of the pseudoaneurysm.

Temporary balloon occlusions are generally performed with the patient awake with a minimum amount of sedation to allow for accurate neurologic evaluation. Neurologic testing should be performed before and after balloon inflation. The duration of balloon occlusion should be for at least 20 minutes, with angiographic confirmation of ICA occlusion. Usually, dual arterial access is needed to evaluate the collateral circulation with the balloon inflated. The patient should be anticoagulated with heparin after guide catheter placement to reduce the risk of a thromboembolic complication.

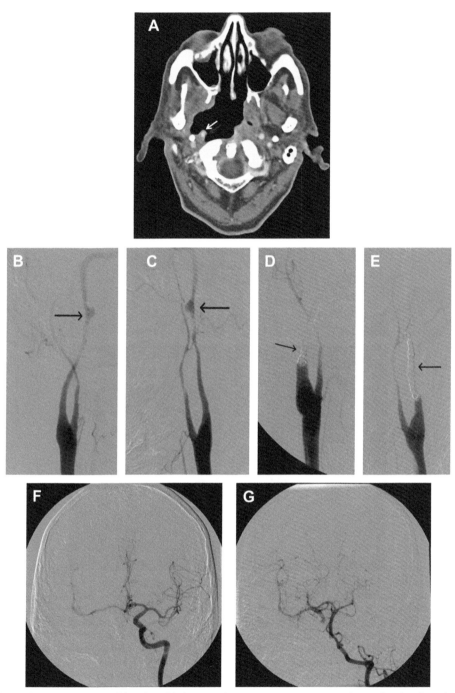

Fig. 2. The patient is a 58-year-old male with laryngeal cancer status post resection, who developed an acute carotid blowout. CT angiography shows a pseudoaneurysm (*white arrow*) of the right internal carotid artery exposed to the post-resection bed (*A*). Cerebral angiography anteroposterior (AP) (*B*) and lateral (*C*) views show a right internal carotid artery pseudoaneurysm (*B*) treated with coil embolization. AP and lateral views of the common carotid artery (*D* and *E*) show occlusion of the right internal carotid artery (*black arrow*). Injection of the left internal carotid artery (*F*) and left vertebral artery (*G*) shows collateral flow to the right internal carotid artery distribution from a patent anterior communicating artery and the right posterior communicating artery.

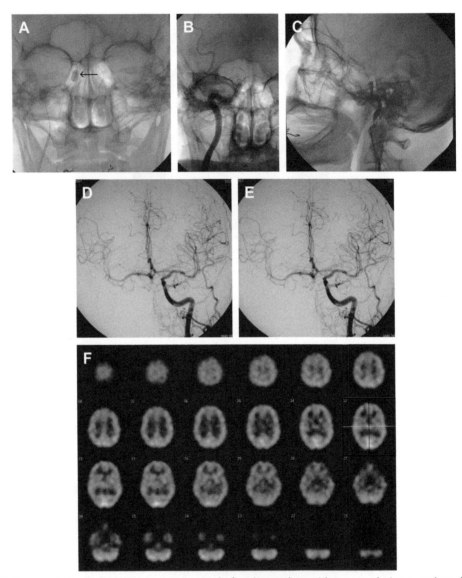

Fig. 3. Balloon occlusion testing is an important test before internal carotid artery occlusion to reduce the risk of stroke. Arterial access is obtained in both femoral arteries. After performance of a diagnostic angiogram, a 5-Fr guide catheter is placed in the internal carotid artery. The patient is heparinized. At our institution, a hyperform balloon (*black arrow*) is advanced into the cavernous internal carotid artery and inflated under roadmap guidance (*A*). Contrast is injected into the guide catheter to confirm vessel occlusion (*B* and *C*). If the patient is neurologically stable with the balloon inflated for 5 to 10 minutes, 99mTc HMPAO is injected for SPECT scanning. The contralateral carotid artery and a vertebral artery are selected to confirm the angiographic presence of adequate collaterals (*D* and *E*). If the patient is neurologically stable, the balloon is deflated after 30 minutes of total occlusion, and then taken for SPECT imaging, which in this case shows symmetric flow bilaterally (*F*).

Balloons that can be used for a temporary balloon occlusion include the Meditech 5 or 7 French Balloon occlusion catheter (Boston Scientific, Meditech, Watertown, MA) or a Hyperform (EV3 Neurovascular, Irvine, CA) 7 × 7-mm balloon. The hyperform balloon is placed just proximal to the ophthalmic artery in the cavernous segment of the carotid artery, if possible. Some operators have used Swan Ganz catheters. Latex balloons can have higher radial force and should be avoided. Regardless of which balloon is used, the balloon should be placed and inflated under roadmap guidance.

Imaging modalities to measure relative or absolute cerebral blood flow (CBF) have been proposed to increase the yield of a temporary balloon occlusion test. The purpose of these measurements is to identify the subset of patients with critical reductions in CBF that are not clinically symptomatic. There are good data that these patients are at higher risk of stroke after sacrifice than the remaining asymptomatic patients with normal flow.[18] Commonly used modalities include 99mTC HMPAO SPECT imaging or CT perfusion scans, either with xenon or contrast administration. HMPAO injection can be performed with the patient on the angiography suite, about 5 minutes after the balloon is inflated. CT perfusion imaging can be a viable alternative; however, this requires transportation of the patient with the balloon in the internal carotid artery from the angiography suite to a CT scanner. Mathis and colleagues[19] reported a 3.2% complication rate with this technique. Their technique involved a 15-minute clinical test occlusion followed by transportation to the CT scanner with the balloon deflated. The balloon is re-inflated in the CT scanner.

These tests can identify an intermediate group of patients who pass the clinical occlusion test but have asymmetric flow on imaging. These patients may require a flow study without balloon occlusion to test for baseline defects. Because the 99mTC HMPAO SPECT scan can be performed with the occlusion balloon removed, and with the radiotracer injected while the balloon can be carefully monitored in the angiography suite, 99mTC HMPAO SPECT is our imaging adjunct of choice.

Hypotensive challenge has also been proposed to improve the yield of a temporary balloon occlusion. A decrease in blood pressure, usually 25% to 33% below baseline can be achieved using a variety of agents including nitroprusside drip, nicardipine drip, or labetolol. A hypotensive challenge should be performed only with careful arterial blood pressure monitoring and with personnel skilled in the adjustment of the medication being used to lower blood pressure. The usual duration of the hypotensive challenge is about 20 minutes.

In patients who are not able to cooperate with neurologic examination, EEG monitoring can be used. Abud and colleagues[20] have advocated the use of delayed venous phase for determining the adequacy of collateral circulation. The advantage of this technique is the ability to perform it under anesthesia. In emergent situations that preclude awake testing, the finding of symmetric venous phases after balloon inflation in the target

carotid artery is very reassuring that sacrifice will be tolerated.

TREATMENT OPTIONS

Decisions regarding treatment options depend on the location and nature of the underlying arterial lesion, as well as the clinical presentation of the patient. Patients with an exposed carotid artery, tumor invasion of the carotid artery, or a nonhemorrhagic pseudoaneurysm can be managed with a scheduled test balloon occlusion, and then internal carotid artery sacrifice if they pass the balloon occlusion test. Patients who fail the balloon occlusion test may benefit from a stent or surgical treatment with vascular bypass.

In patients with an acute carotid blowout or a sentinel hemorrhage, distinguishing involvement of the ECA versus ICA or CCA can be very important for treatment, and is likely to be a major reason for improved outcomes with endovascular versus surgical therapy. Patients in whom only an abnormal tumor blush is noted can be managed with ECA branch embolization only, and patients in whom the bleeding source or pseudoaneurysm is clearly identified as originating in the external carotid artery selective vessel occlusion by endovascular means (coils, liquid embolic agents) can be performed without disrupting the internal or common carotid artery (see **Fig. 1**), which will have a higher complication rate.

In patients in whom the bleeding source originates in the internal or common carotid artery, treatment options include vessel occlusion (see **Fig. 2**) and endovascular remodeling strategies with a stent (**Fig. 4**). In patients with an acute carotid blowout or a sentinel bleed, a formal balloon occlusion test cannot be performed. For these patients, if the patient is stable enough, an angiographic assessment of collateral flow can be made, with or without evaluation of venous phase asymmetry after placement of a proximal balloon occlusion catheter. Internal or common carotid artery lesions in these patients can be treated with ICA occlusion. If there is a concern for poor collateral flow and CTA evaluation showed good soft tissue coverage of the involved artery, endovascular remodeling strategies with a stent may be used.

General Guidelines

In the setting of an acute hemorrhage, general anesthesia and critical care expertise is an absolute must. These patients may become hemodynamically unstable and the procedure is often undertaken in concert with resuscitation efforts. Do not wear your best shoes. Anesthesia is

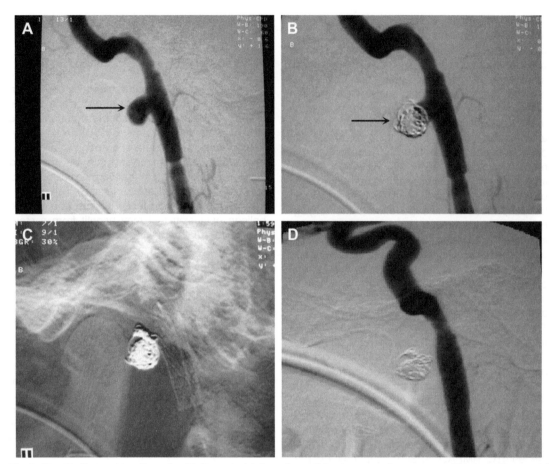

Fig. 4. Stent/coil reconstruction of a high cervical internal carotid artery pseudoaneurysm. This is a 47-year-old man 7 days status post oropharyngeal resection of an squamous cell carcinoma with a radial artery pedicle flap reconstruction. He suffered massive arterial bleeding through the nose and mouth while driving from home from the hospital. (*A*) Diagnostic angiography of the left common carotid artery shows a left internal carotid artery pseudoaneurysm (*black arrow*). A 6-mm × 2-cm SMART stent was placed across the aneurysm neck. (*B*) The pseudoaneurysm was successfully coiled with detachable coils (*black arrow*), with a small residual neck. (*C*) An anatomic image shows the relationship of the stent and coils. (*D*) Follow-up angiogram 48 hours later shows complete occlusion of the aneurysm, with no residual neck, from the flow-directing effects of the stent. This patient remains well now 8 years after the procedure.

needed for several reasons, including adequate airway control (often in the setting of active oral bleeding), sedation, and paralytic agents. All are required for safe and effective endovascular therapy. Large-bore intravenous lines or central lines are important for resuscitation efforts. A large peripheral arterial sheath is important for accommodating the balloon occlusion catheters often required for proximal control. A second site for arterial access is often needed.

Permanent Internal Carotid Artery Occlusion

The basic principles of proximal and distal control remain paramount in vessel sacrifice for carotid blowout syndrome. The first goal, once carotid sacrifice is selected as the therapeutic maneuver, is to achieve proximal flow control. In general this is accomplished with a balloon occlusion catheter such as the Meditech (Boston Scientific) or Merci (Concentric Medical, Mountain View, CA) catheters.[21] We use little or no pressurized flush through the central bore of the catheter after inflating the occlusion balloon, as this may allow clots or debris to flow into the cranial circulation. Some back bleeding is fine. Once the balloon is inflated under roadmap control, we will often confirm occlusion with a very gentle injection of contrast material. A roadmap of the carotid can be obtained. We then advance a microcatheter carefully beyond the site of vessel injury. Alternatively, if the lesion does not allow antegrade navigation, the internal carotid beyond the lesion can often be occluded in a retrograde fashion via the anterior or posterior communicating arteries. This retrograde approach usually requires general anesthesia and a second site of arterial access. For antegrade procedures, after deploying 1 to 2 detachable coils, the embolization is completed with 10 or more pushable fibered coils, such as Cook Tornado coils (Cook, Bloomington, IL). Liquid embolics, such as ethyl vinyl copolymer or Onyx (EV3 Neurovascular) can be used as an adjunct to coils. This can be a very effective means of immediately eliminating back flow from the distal internal carotid artery in emergent situations. Detachable balloons also have a role. These may return to the market in the future. Once the distal occlusion has been accomplished, attention can be turned to the proximal segment. Placement of coils across the ruptured segment should be avoided for the risk of infection. This cannot always be avoided owing to the length of the vessel. The information from the CT study can be useful in determining the length and location of exposed vessel. The proximal occlusion is generally obtained with coils, but as above, liquid agents and potentially detachable balloons may have a role as well.

If possible, patients who undergo an internal carotid artery occlusion should not be heparinized before proximal control has been obtained. Decisions regarding the use of antiplatelet medications or anticoagulation after the procedure should be made based on the perceived potential for distal embolization. For example, there is no reason for these medications after sacrifice of branches of the ECA. Patients who have undergone permanent carotid occlusion should be followed closely in an ICU setting with careful monitoring of blood pressure and hydration. The patient should be maintained in a recumbent position initially with gradual mobilization over a 24- to 48-hour period.

Internal Carotid Artery Preservation with Stents

Although permanent occlusion of the internal carotid artery is an effective treatment for carotid blowout syndrome, the risk of stroke associated with this technique, particularly when temporary balloon occlusion to assess collateral circulation cannot be performed, has led to efforts to find alternative treatments for patients with carotid blowout syndrome. When there is concern that the patient cannot tolerate sacrifice of the internal carotid artery, endovascular remodeling techniques can be effective treatments for carotid blowout. Stent-assisted endovascular reconstruction of the carotid artery is an evolving therapy for lesions

that involve the internal carotid artery. Therapeutic options include placement of a covered stent across the lesion, stent-assisted coiling, or placement of overlapping bare metal stents across the carotid artery for flow re-direction.

Bare metal stents, with or without coils in the pseudoaneurysm, are likely less effective in the short term than vessel sacrifice (see **Fig. 4**). Examples of covered stents that can be used include the Wallgraft stent, Jo-Stent, and the Niti-S stent. Covered stent placement such as the Wallgraft stent requires favorable anatomic factors such as ability to place a 9- or 10-Fr vascular sheath, relatively straight artery, and lack of proximal stenoses. In addition, other disadvantages of covered stent placement include the need to maintain patients on aspirin and plavix, and reports of infection or delayed complications such as stent extrusion in patients treated by endovascular reconstruction techniques for carotid blowout syndrome.[11,22–24]

External Carotid Artery Lesions

Pseudoaneurysms of the external carotid artery can be treated with endovascular coiling (see **Fig. 1**), or permanent obstruction with liquid embolics such as glue. In some series, lesions of the external carotid artery are more common than lesions of the internal or common carotid arteries. Bleeding from a head and neck tumor can often be treated with temporary agents such as polyvinyl alcohol particles.[25]

COMPLICATIONS/OUTCOMES
Stroke

Abrupt occlusion of the internal carotid artery without provocative testing is associated with a substantial risk of stroke, up to 50%.[12,16] Prior temporary balloon occlusion with clinical testing and other adjuncts such as perfusion imaging, or provocative testing such as hypotensive challenge reduce this rate. Endovascular remodeling techniques are also a way to lower the risk of stroke from abrupt carotid occlusion when feasible. Stroke may also occur during embolization of external carotid artery lesions.

Infection

There are case reports of brain abscesses developing after stent graft placement for treatment of carotid blowout syndrome, presumably because deployment of a stent graft in a field that is undergoing radiation necrosis can result in foreign body contamination.[23] In our own experience, we have seen one patient develop brain abscesses after sacrifice, likely from septic emboli occurring at the site of the arterial wall breakdown as a consequence of the communication with the nasopharynx.

Recurrent Carotid Blowout Syndrome

Chaloupka and colleagues[26] defined recurrent carotid blowout syndrome as a sentinel hemorrhage or acute carotid blowout within 12 hours of treatment of a previous carotid blowout syndrome and any patient who developed an exposed carotid artery at any time after treatment for carotid blowout syndrome. In their series, 26% of patients had recurrent bleeding. Recurrent bleeding could be attributed to either progressive disease, such as wound dehiscence, flap necrosis, or treatment failure (recurrent bleeding from the same site that had been treated by endovascular or surgical means).

Stent Extrusion

There are case reports of stent extrusion resulting in stroke or rebleeding in patients treated by endovascular means for carotid blowout syndrome, highlighting the instability of the arterial wall in patients with head and neck tumors treated with radiation therapy, and in patients at high risk of developing infections in the treatment bed. The struts of the stent may predispose to erosion of the vessel wall at the edges of the stent.[24,27]

OUTCOMES

Surgical therapy for carotid blowout syndrome has been associated with a 60% neurologic morbidity and 40% mortality. Reported case series data with endovascular treatment has reported substantially better outcomes, with initial reports having greater than 80% survival and much lower neurologic morbidity (0% immediate postprocedure ischemic events in two case series by Chaloupka and colleagues)[8,9] from endovascular treatment for carotid blowout syndrome.[4]

The rate of recurrent bleeding after endovascular therapy may be as high as 26%.[11]

The available case report data from stent placement for carotid blowout syndrome indicates that although such a strategy may be very effective for acute treatment, stent placement may not be an effective long-term strategy.[24,27]

SUMMARY

The endovascular management of carotid blowout syndrome is a potentially life-saving intervention. Advances in CT angiography have made it easier to accurately localize lesions and guide endovascular treatment. At present, vessel sacrifice is the most commonly used and most effective strategy. Depending on the urgency of the clinical situation, some assessment of collateral flow should be performed. Vessel-preserving approaches are less well established and currently carry long-term risks of infection or stent extrusion. In some cases, however, these are preferred.

REFERENCES

1. Vokes EE, Weischelbaum RR, Lippman SM, et al. Head and neck cancer. N Engl J Med 1993;328(3): 184–94.
2. Medina, Jesus. Neck dissection. In: Bailey BJ, Johnson JT, Newlands SD, editors. Head and neck surgery—otolaryngology. New York: Lippincott Williams and Wilkins; 2006. p. 1585–609.
3. Haddad RI, Shin DM. Recent advances in head and neck cancer. N Engl J Med 2008;359(11):1143–54.
4. Maran AG, Amin M, Wilson JA. Radical neck dissection: a 19-year experience. J Laryngol Otol 1989; 103(8):760–4.
5. Katras T, Baltazar U, Colvett K, et al. Radiation-related arterial disease. Am Surg 1999;65(12):1176–9.
6. Borsany SJ. Rupture of the carotids following radical neck surgery in irradiated patients. Ear Nose Throat J 1962;41:531–3.
7. Ketcham AS, Hoye RC. Spontaneous carotid artery hemorrhage after head and neck surgery. Am J Surg 1965;110:649–55.
8. Chaloupka JC, Putnam CM, Citardi MJ, et al. Endovascular therapy for the carotid blowout syndrome in head and neck surgical patients: diagnostic and managerial considerations. AJNR Am J Neuroradiol 1996;17(5):843–52.
9. Citardi MJ, Chaloupka JC, Son YH, et al. Management of carotid artery rupture by monitored endovascular therapeutic occlusion (1988–1994). Laryngoscope 1995;105:1086–92.
10. Cohen J, Rad I. Contemporary management of carotid blowout. Curr Opin Otolaryngol Head Neck Surg 2004;12(2):110–5.
11. Lesly WS, Chaloupka JC, Weigele JB, et al. Preliminary experience with endovascular reconstruction for the management of carotid blowout syndrome. AJNR Am J Neuroradiol 2003;24(5):975–81.
12. Nishioka H. Report on the cooperative study of intracranial aneurysms and subarachnoid hemorrhage, VIII. Part I: results of the treatment of intracranial aneurysms by occlusion of the carotid artery in the neck. J Neurosurg 1966;25:660–82.
13. Winn HR, Richardson AE, Jane JA. Late morbidity and mortality of common carotid ligation for posterior communicating aneurysms: a comparison to conservative treatment. J Neurosurg 1977;47(5): 727–36.

14. de Vries EJ, Sekhar LN, Horton JA, et al. A new method to predict safe resection of the internal carotid artery. Laryngoscope 1990;100(1):85–8.

15. Gonzalez CF, Moret J. Balloon occlusion of the carotid artery prior to surgery for neck tumors. AJNR Am J Neuroradiol 1990;11(4):649–52.

16. Linskey ME, Jungreis CA, Yonas H, et al. Stroke risk after abrupt internal carotid artery sacrifice: accuracy of preoperative assessment with balloon test occlusion and stable xenon enhanced CT. AJNR Am J Neuroradiol 1994;15(5):829–43.

17. Eckard DA, Purdy PD, Bonte FJ. Temporary balloon occlusion of the carotid artery combined with brain blood flow imaging as a test to predict tolerance prior to permanent carotid sacrifice. AJNR Am J Neuroradiol 1992;13(6):1565–9.

18. Marshall RS, Lazar RA, Young WL, et al. Clinical utility of quantitative cerebral blood flow measurement during internal carotid artery test occlusions. Neurosurgery 2002;50(5):996–1005.

19. Mathis JM, Barr JD, Jungreis CA, et al. Temporary balloon test occlusion of the internal carotid artery: experience in 500 cases. AJNR Am J Neuroradiol 1995;16(4):749–54.

20. Abud DG, Spelle L, Piotin M, et al. Venous phase timing during balloon test occlusion as a criterion for permanent internal carotid artery sacrifice. AJNR Am J Neuroradiol 2005;26:2602–9.

21. Graves VB, Perl J, Strother CM, et al. Endovascular occlusion of the carotid or vertebral artery with temporary proximal flow arrest and microcoil: clinical results. AJNR Am J Neuroradiol 1997;18:1201–6.

22. Kim HS, Lee DH, Kim HJ, et al. Life threatening common carotid blowout: rescue treatment with a newly designed self expanding covered nitinol stent. Br J Radiol 2006;79:226–31.

23. Chang FC, Lirng JF, Tai SK, et al. Brain abscess formation: a delayed complication of carotid blowout syndrome treated by self expandable stent graft. AJNR Am J Neuroradiol 2006;27(7):1543–5.

24. Simental A, Johnson Jonas, Horowitz M. Delayed complications of endovascular stenting for carotid blowout. Am J Otol 2003;24(6):417–9.

25. Luo CB, Teng MM, Chang FC, et al. Transarterial embolization of acute external carotid blowout syndrome with profuse oronasal bleeding by N-butyl-cyanoacrylate. Am J Emerg Med 2006;24(6):702–8.

26. Chaloupka JC, Roth TC, Putnam CM, et al. Recurrent carotid blowout syndrome: diagnostic and therapeutic challenges in a newly recognized subgroup of patients. AJNR Am J Neuroradiol 1999;20(6):1069–77.

27. Pyun HW, Lee DH, Yoo HM, et al. Placement of covered stents for carotid blowout in patients with head and neck cancer: follow up results after rescue treatments. AJNR Am J Neuroradiol 2007;28(8):1594–7.

Index

Note: Page numbers of article titles are in **boldface** type.

Moving?

Make sure your subscription moves with you!

To notify us of your new address, find your **Clinics Account Number** (located on your mailing label above your name), and contact customer service at:

E-mail: elspcs@elsevier.com

800-654-2452 (subscribers in the U.S. & Canada)
314-453-7041 (subscribers outside of the U.S. & Canada)

Fax number: 314-523-5170

Elsevier Periodicals Customer Service
11830 Westline Industrial Drive
St. Louis, MO 63146

*To ensure uninterrupted delivery of your subscription, please notify us at least 4 weeks in advance of move.

Printed and bound by CPI Group (UK) Ltd, Croydon, CR0 4YY

03/10/2024

01040361-0015